Praise for
Aging Forward

T0253120

"David and Martha Dunkelman's important book about aging affects every American by addressing this critical question: How can more Americans age in health and dignity in their own homes or in places designed better to meet their needs for care and community? Both policy makers and concerned citizens can use their ideas to implement changes we all know we need."

—Hillary Rodham Clinton

"The history of long-term care for older persons is filled with mistakes and shortsighted solutions. The hopeful message of this book is that change is possible. Tomorrow's seniors will be the beneficiaries of new digital technologies that will significantly improve their ability to live independent and dignified lives."

—Stephen Golant, Ph.D., *Professor Emeritus, University of Florida, and author of* Aging in the Right Place

"*Aging Forward* is full of insightful, provocative, and innovative ideas that will help move forward the national debate about the much-needed reform of the patchwork of healthcare for older adults.... A must read for anyone who cares about improving the healthcare of older adults."

—Thomas J. Fairchild, Ph.D., *Adjunct Associate Professor, Departments of Behavioral Health & Health Services and Internal Medicine & Geriatrics, The University of North Texas Health Science Center at Fort Worth*

"This groundbreaking book highlights the impact of the deluge of older people on our broken healthcare system [and] offers a realistic and practical path out of the current stagnation and denial."

—Richard Berman, *Former Director, Office of Health Systems Management, New York State*

"This groundbreaking book envisions a new direction for aging and aging care networks."

—Nancy J. Smyth, Ph.D., LCSW, *Professor and Former Dean, University at Buffalo School of Social Work*

Aging
Forward

A New Path for Health, Technology, and Community

by

David M. Dunkelman, J.D., M.S.

and

Martha Dunkelman, Ph.D.

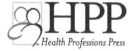
HPP
Health Professions Press

Baltimore • London • Sydney

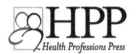

Health Professions Press, Inc.
Post Office Box 10624
Baltimore, Maryland 21285-0624

Copyright © 2023 by David and Martha Dunkelman.
All rights reserved.

Interior and cover designs by Erin Geoghegan.

Typeset and manufactured in the United States of America by
Books International, Dulles, Virginia.

Library of Congress Cataloging-in-Publication Data
Names: Dunkelman, David M., author. | Dunkelman, Martha, author.
Title: Aging forward : a new path for health, technology, and community /
    by David M. Dunkelman, J.D., M.S. and Martha Dunkelman, Ph.D.
Description: Baltimore, Maryland : Health Professions Press, [2023] |
    Includes bibliographical references and index.
Identifiers: LCCN 2023002432 (print) | LCCN 2023002433 (ebook) |
    ISBN 9781956801033 (paperback) | ISBN 9781956801040 (epub)
Subjects: LCSH: Older people--Services for. | Aging--Social aspects.
Classification: LCC HV1451 .D856 2023 (print) | LCC HV1451 (ebook) |
    DDC 362.6--dc23/eng/20230119
LC record available at https://lccn.loc.gov/2023002432
LC ebook record available at https://lccn.loc.gov/2023002433

British Library Cataloguing in Publication data are available from the British Library.

Contents

Our increased longevity is having an epochal impact on how we live and on our gender roles, generational balance, retirement financing, healthcare expenses, and government spending.

Medical, sociological, psychological, environmental, and economic changes mean that the much-improved lives of older adults no longer reflect our outdated conceptions of aging.

The traditional nursing home was built for a population entirely different from today's older adults, and our care models are no longer suited to the chronic conditions or profound frailty of those served.

Creating an entirely new nursing home design revealed that the behaviors, sights, sounds, and smells of traditional care settings are not actually the result of aging, but artifacts of an inappropriate delivery system.

The traditional, highly specialized Industrial Era healthcare
system we have is a barrier to the optimal functioning of the
Law of Interchangeable Interventions. The Digital Age offers an
alternative that engages all the assets and resources available
for deployment in the United States.

Just as digital technology has dramatically changed other
sectors of industry in the United States, it will also transform
aging and healthcare. A hypothetical model demonstrates
the revolutionary possibilities in how and where care for older
people is delivered.

Digitization will be an accelerant for the Law of Interchangeable
Interventions, radically changing the direction and shape of each
component of the "continuum of care" available to older adults.

A new networked care system will offer both new solutions
and new challenges. The nation's regulatory regime must be
refashioned to address the challenges.

Integration of frail older adults into communities will not be
blocked or paralyzed because it will settle naturally into the
rhythm of modern life in the United States.

Profound frailty correlated with age will cease to drive people
into segregated institutions, and these people will remain
integrated into our communities, thereby recasting leadership,
the communities themselves, and the possibilities for aging.

Contents

About the Authors

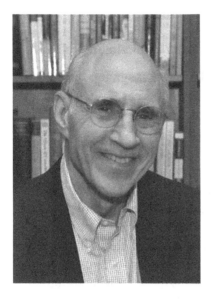

David Dunkelman, M.S., J.D.

Raised in Ohio, David Dunkelman expanded his experience by traveling around the world for a year after graduating from college. He visited 26 countries and three war zones, and observed many ways people live and die. He left the United States an angry young man and returned a patriot after seeing how so many other societies functioned. After graduating from Temple University School of Law, he helped his family's apparel company grow to an organization distributing to 5,000 retailers nationally. The company closed when computers suddenly disrupted the nation's centuries-old clothing supply chain, an ominous preview to what would also happen to aging in America.

Changing focus, Dunkelman earned a master's degree from the Center for Studies in Aging at the University of North Texas, after which he eventually landed in Buffalo, New York, where for 30 years he was the founding President and CEO of The Harry and Jeanette Weinberg Campus, one of the nation's largest and most multifaceted campuses for older people. The campus was the first such organization to be named a winner of the national Peter F. Drucker Award for Innovation in Nonprofit Management.

Among his many individual awards are the Community Leadership Award from the Foundation for Jewish Philanthropies, Buffalo

(2013), and the Dr. Evan Calkins Meritorious Service Award for "life-time contributions to the field of aging," presented by the Western New York Network in Aging, Inc. (2007).

Using creative problem-solving techniques developed at the State University of New York at Buffalo, Dunkelman has consulted nationally with more than 25 communities, helping them to develop strategic approaches to facility and programmatic design for older people. He writes and speaks about aging in America.

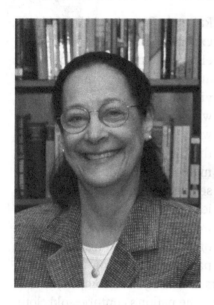

Martha Dunkelman, Ph.D.

Martha Dunkelman is a writer and editor who has written numerous articles, reviews, and brochures, as well as serving as book editor for an online periodical. She has also written and edited materials for the Educational Testing Service and the College Board. She credits her father, Dr. Maurice Levine, with teaching her to write in her teenage years, when she was not always the most willing student.

A graduate of Wellesley College, she later received a doctorate from New York University under the wise and kind guidance of H. W. Janson and spent many years in teaching and administration as a professor at Wright State University, the University at Buffalo, and Canisius College.

She learned about the care of older people from decades of bearing witness to the struggles and achievements of her husband David.

Acknowledgments

We shared the experiences described in this narrative with many friends, colleagues, advisors, and mentors. They all contributed to the attempt to capture America's aging over the past 50 years and project it forward. Their gifts were cumulative, and we thank them for shaping our understanding.

This book was born from conversations with Judson Mead, whose ideas helped to crystallize some of the most difficult concepts about the aging experience in America that David was witnessing directly. Without his questions, clear thinking, and written contributions, this book would never have come into existence.

The foundations for the observations and analysis offered in the book were laid in earlier years by several beloved teachers and guides:

Alan S. Engel, Ph.D., college advisor and supporter for over 55 years

Jerry D. Smart,* M.S., J.D., David Glaser,* and Gerald N. Cohen,* M.S.W., internship preceptors in long-term care administration

Monsignor Charles J. Fahey, who guided me towards and along the way

Bert Hayslip Jr., Ph.D., Professor Emeritus of Lifespan Development Psychology at North Texas State University (now the University of North Texas), who taught a course that influenced the entire career that followed

Thomas J. Fairchild, Ph.D., thesis adviser, lifelong collaborator, and lifelong friend

Herbert Shore,* Ed.D., teacher, mentor, and profound inspiration

---

*Of blessed memory.

At the campus in Buffalo, David was part of an extraordinary group of collaborators:

A caring, devoted, forward-thinking Board of Directors

Ten board chairs with whom David was able to share sensitive personal and organizational hopes and fears; five of them— Herbert Mennen, Hyman Polakoff,* CPA, Ambassador Leonard Rochwarger,* John Greenberger, M.B.A., and Kenneth A. Rogers, M.B.A.—worked through particular pivotal moments in the life of the campus

Peter Fleischmann, true asset of Buffalo's Jewish community

Samuel L. Shapiro, Esq., who protected the campus through torturous legal terrain

Arnold Maxick, CPA, who guided us through continual financial gauntlets

Robert Mayer, M.B.A., CFO, financial ballast, who became CEO upon David's retirement

Randi Dressel, M.B.A., COO, hour-to-hour partner in administration who devoted decades of her life to operating the campus

Amy Hashemi, L.M.S.W., M.B.A., Judith R. Katz, Diane Koteras, and Dana Notaro, who led our magnificent staff in caring for our thousands of residents, patients, clients, participants, and their families

Nathan Benderson,* whose insights made him a most unforgettable person in David's career, and the Benderson family

Randy Benderson, who guided the construction and expansion of the Campus

Professional expertise and leadership came from:

Lorraine G. Hiatt, Ph.D., brilliant conceptualizer of environments for older people

Zachary Rosenfeld,* AIA, who reconstructed nursing home life

Community collaborators included:

Ann F. Monroe and the Health Foundation for Western and Central New York

Pamela Krawczyk-Greene, M.S., Mary Pruski, RN, Kathleen M. Flynn, M.B.A., and Tracy Van Patten Sawicki, fellowship team

partners at the Health Foundation for Western and Central
New York

Virginia Oehler, M.A., Fellowship Director

The John R. Oishei Foundation

Diane R. Bessel, M.S.W., Ph.D., consultant and partner at the Town
Square for Aging

New York State Senator Mary Lou Rath and New York State
Assemblyman Robin Schimminger, J.D., stalwart advocates on
behalf of aging programs

Louis P. Ciminelli

State and national collaborators included:

The New York State Department of Health

The Harry and Jeanette Weinberg Foundation

Paula Wilson, D.S.W.

Suggestions and improvements to the manuscript came from:

Mary Magnus and Linda Francis, our editors; Kaitlin Konecke,
our marketing manager; and the entire team at Health
Professions Press, whose unerring judgment and continual
encouragement brought this work to the light of day

Richard R. Hurtig, Ph.D., with whom David spent many an evening batting around ideas and who helped frame the entire
manuscript

Paul Pevsner, M.D., who provided companionship and confidence
through the book's long gestation

Robert W. Buechner, Esq., Barbara Bunker, Ph.D., Sara Caples,
AIA, Thomas J. Fairchild, Ph.D., Peter Fleischmann, Peter
Gold, Ph.D., John Greenberger, Lito Gutierrez, M.D., Judith
Hurtig, Ph.D., Debra Pincus, Ph.D., Sam Radin, Esq., and
Michael Skaff

And most of all:

Marc and Anna, our wonderful and tolerant son and daughter,
whose childhoods were saturated with the community aging
enterprise

Special thanks to Anna and husband Geoff Gallagher who
helped create the word "benesence," to Marc and his wife

Kathryn, who provided endless encouragement and support, and to granddaughters Emilia and Helen, who give us joy and hope for the future

And to each other, we say, with the love of more than 50 years together, "A book about all of it? Who could have imagined it would come to this?"

Welcome

This is our story. This is your story.

If you're holding this book or viewing a screen, and if you live in the United States, this book is about you. It is not a metaphor, a parable, an allegory, or a moral lesson; nor is it an exhortation to take some political action. It is about your future, a future that is being shaped by how you think and live right now.

Unlike other books on the market that decry the current problems and expenses of caring for older adults, this one describes how the experience of growing old will transform in the coming years into a phase of life that is much better than it has ever been before. It looks into the factors that make this transformation possible and at some of the barriers that may slow it down. In the process, it explains how our view of aging has changed since the 1960s or so, and how it will now change again. We will burst through the chrysalis created to address infectious disease in the Industrial Age and fly into communities to address chronic conditions in the Digital Age.

My approach in this book entwines both my personal experience and the history of aging in this country in order to show how seemingly disparate phenomena are interconnected. Aging, particularly *frail* aging, must be understood as a totality of many factors. The Digital Age's new processing power will enable us to gather and sort, analyze, and synthesize all the components and to integrate even profound frail aging into 21st-century life in the United States.

For reasons described in this book, many have been denied the opportunity to include aging in their interest sets. Even cursory discussions of one of the most fascinating personal and societal stories in our lives are all too rare. I am cognizant of the layers of denial around aging and of the inaccurate and unfortunate accumulations residing within us. I have attempted to find a way to entice you to add aging to your ongoing interests. If aging becomes a subject of interest in people's lives, the world will change for people of all ages.

No one has told this exciting and interesting story before. And we will be better off if we can see the transformation coming and prepare for it.

Most important is the new and surprising message of this book: We need not be afraid of our future selves. By describing what is happening all around us and understanding how we got here, we can get a clearer view of where we are going. Aging can be an opening to decades of your life that you need not fear, ones that offer their own bounties to savor. Although it has its own complement of difficulties, as does every era of life, older age is an era that can be, and for most of us will be, very different from what we anticipate.

Well into my 70s myself as I wrote this book, I will tell you in my own voice how I have been continually discovering the world of aging. This is a story of the evolution of the field and of my own thinking about it. I hope my process will help you understand yours. Welcome.

Note: Martha and David Dunkelman wrote this book as a collaboration. However, because the experiences recounted are those of David alone, we have made the joint decision to use the first person singular in the text.

Dedicated to

Henri Parens
Guide, Teacher, Role Model, Hero

"There is an epidemic failure within the game to understand what is really happening."

Peter Brandt, *Moneyball*, the movie

Introduction

We have all had some experience with the nursing homes of today and have felt fear and anxiety from what we have seen of their sights and smells, their long corridors with limp figures in wheelchairs waiting for help, their gloomy hospital atmosphere. In a later chapter, I will try to explain how these facilities have come to be so awful. But first, let me show you a picture of how aging is going to be soon, in the course of our lifetimes. After that, I will backtrack to explain what is going on at present, and then we will all be ready to see the future in detail.

Mrs. Smith's Story

It is 5 or 10 years from now. Mrs. Smith is 93 years old, with chronic arthritis, high blood pressure, diabetes, and significant hearing loss. Frail as she may seem, she lives contentedly in her home of many years. She is surrounded by unobtrusive devices that make it possible for her to remain safely and comfortably in her own familiar environment, with access to more personalized care if she needs it and to social activities of her own choosing.

This may sound like a dream or a picture of the distant future, but, as we will see, it is a scenario that is being made possible through digital technology and intelligent planning. Mrs. Smith wears a thin wrist monitor. Her bed and many of her kitchen and bathroom appliances are connected to a data-collection service that can monitor her heart function, weight, blood pressure, glucose level, and whatever else is needed. Her pill boxes open automatically with a beep that sounds in her hearing aids so that she doesn't miss it. Food, medicine, household needs, a ride, and a helping hand are all easily available with a click or a call on her phone or tablet. Nurses and other helpers visit throughout the day on a schedule, with extra visits when necessary.

As Mrs. Smith's capacities diminish, adjustments to medications, food preparation, physical therapy, and companionship are made in consultation with Mrs. Smith herself, as well as her family and her caregivers. Cameras can be activated for check-ins and casual conversations. Entertainment and socialization are available both at home and elsewhere. A multichannel television can stream lectures and live discussions. Rides to social events are arranged remotely, and emergency help can arrive within minutes. Mrs. Smith is relaxed and happy to be in the home she knows, with her own dishes and books and pillows. Her loving and anxious daughter, whether at home across town or on vacation at the beach, can follow along the path of her mother's day and still get to work or childcare on time.

Today, a frail older resident in a traditional nursing home has an adjustable bed surrounded by an array of services from a call button to a table on wheels. In the new era, the frail person, in his or her own dwelling, like our fictional Mrs. Smith, will have his or her own familiar bed, with a phone or tablet within reach that will allow the person to obtain many of the same services that using the call button provided, from ordering meals to calling for an aide. Data collected from myriad devices will be monitored and orchestrated by systems and selected people who will see when interventions and adjustments need to be made. When an aide comes in, it is likely that the person is someone with whom the client is compatible. The data will be available to family members designated by the client, who will be able to see how their older relative is doing physically, track his or her activities of daily living, and observe how much the loved one is participating in various social activities.

Similar features will be available if adults decide, for one reason or another, to leave their private homes for a place that is purpose-built for older adults. These settings will already incorporate features designed to make life easier. The physical environment will be reshaped and retooled to calibrate the losses correlated with chronological age and ameliorate physical deficiencies. Walking distances will be shorter, lighting will be adjusted for changing vision and to combat depression, and carpets will be chosen to reduce falls. Color and furniture will maximize safety and minimize confusion. The environment will accommodate the person as his or her capabilities shrink.

Assistive accommodations can be camouflaged. The specially adapted flooring, faucets, toilets, lights, and handrails will not have a geriatric look. They will not mark the inhabitants as old. When the assistive environment is designed to look like any other, the conditions encourage the people living there to respond accordingly. Masking the props and mechanisms that keep a person upright takes away the constant reminders of incapacity. If we could build all our nursing homes from scratch today, we would build them to look like apartments, and the people they housed would not look as lost as those living in many nursing homes today.

We have the technology now to achieve this dignified and individualized life for the frail older members of our society. With the help of computer programmers and algorithms, we can solve many of the problems around aging care that worry us, even the threat of skyrocketing costs. We need to allow the natural workings of a phenomenon I call the Law of Interchangeable Interventions, which affirms that people who are given the freedom to make their own decisions will choose the least expensive, least medicalized, and least invasive way to solve a problem. Then the world of aging will change for the better. Older adults will become part of our communities rather than isolated and hidden away, and that will benefit us all.

A New Framework to Overcome
Antiquated Stereotypes

As a society we have an underlying uneasiness about the future because we misunderstand the condition of aging in the present. Traditional stereotypes about old age that we learned from our parents and grandparents no longer describe what is happening. Our outdated perspective gives rise to all kinds of unnecessary anxiety about the relationship of aging and healthcare, unmanageable costs, the availability of long-term care, and other problems.

We can, and indeed must, become comfortable with a vision of a new era for older age, that, like Mrs. Smith's, is less institutionalized and more digitally networked. It will also cost less. My hope is that you, the reader, will suspend disbelief long enough to perceive the coming transformation. I believe older age has been hidden under layers of outdated stereotypes and responses that have masked its true nature. But now we have the tools to strip away much of the detritus clogging the system.

We have known for a long time that our current framework for older age is not sustainable and that all our attempts to adjust it have been insufficient. The coming transformation that this book describes means that the Baby Boomer generation, born between 1946 and 1964, can expect to live into their 70s, 80s, 90s, and beyond in conditions immeasurably better than those that were available to their parents and grandparents. Revealing the true nature of older age will provide the hope, energy, and confidence to move forward, and will peel away the fears that have inhibited improving our aging care.

Understanding the future of aging is important to adults of all ages. If we have aging parents, we are likely to encounter the care system for older adults. When we grow old ourselves, we will certainly become involved with some version of aging care. Coming generations will pay for, redesign, and operate whatever care system evolves. We will be able to understand better what happens tomorrow if we understand the state of aging as it is today, where it came from, and where it should be going.

PART I

How We Got Here

CHAPTER 1

The New Scale of Aging

To understand why the brave new world for older adults has not yet arrived, it is important to realize how much has changed since the early 20th century. You may not be fully aware of what has changed and the consequences, but these developments made it possible and even imperative to find more economical and feasible arrangements for older adults. We must understand how these changes have transformed our world before we can adjust to them in a realistic and productive manner.

First and foremost, humankind has experienced a sudden, substantial increase in life expectancy. According to population researcher Abdel Omran (1971), "during The Age of Pestilence and Famine [up until the 19th century] . . . the average life expectancy at birth . . . [was] vacillating between 20 and 40 years."[1] Today, except in the least developed and poorest parts of the world, the profile is different. For the first time in human history, almost everyone gets old. Because the change happened suddenly and recently, we haven't recognized its impact.

Of course, there have always been people who lived long lives. Even when life expectancy was 45 years, some people lived to 85. But in 1900 in the United States, only 1 person in every 623 was 85 or older. Today, 1 person in 56 is 85 or older. In 2030, when the Baby Boom generation starts to reach 85, 1 person in 38 will be 85 or older, and by 2050 that number will be 1 in 20.[2] This estimate is based on current mortality rates that do not assume any life-extending breakthroughs in the next 40 years. In just a century and a half, from 1900 to 2050, the 85-year-old has evolved from being a rare occurrence to being a frequent one.

To think of the change another way, in 1900 in the United States, life expectancy at birth was about 45 years for men and 47 years for women. In 2000, life expectancy at birth was about 75 for men and 79 for women. During the 20th century, therefore, life expectancy almost doubled. Since the total population itself increased by 4 times during that period, the number of people 65 and older increased 35 times, from 122,000 to 4,250,000. Individuals 65 and older are actually the fastest-growing segment of the U.S. population.[3]

Two longevity revolutions produced our huge population of older adults. One change affected younger people; the other, strongly influenced by the first, affected older ones.

The First Longevity Revolution

The first longevity revolution is easier to see because it happened entirely in the past, beginning a little more than a century ago. We can look back at it with some perspective.

In the 1970s, Omran proposed a model that led to a similar but broader conclusion about longevity. He divided the epidemiological history of humankind into three ages: the Age of Pestilence and Famine, which occupies most of human history; the Age of Receding Pandemics, roughly 1850–1950 in the United States, when we conquered most infectious diseases; and the Age of Degenerative and Manmade Diseases, such as cardiovascular disease and cancer.[4] In the 50 years since Omran published this scheme, epidemiologists have come to see that we are now living in a fourth age, the Age of Delayed Degenerative Diseases.[5] Most of us now survive infancy, youth, and adulthood thanks to modern sanitation, public health practices, and modern medicine, and we eventually arrive at old age. In the current Age of Delayed Degenerative Disease, we often continue to survive even after we become older. We get more years of life because the onset of degenerative diseases is postponed. The nature of our current experience suggests that we may actually be in a new, fifth epidemiologic era, what I call the Age of Extended Chronic Conditions. It is not just that we have delayed the onset of degenerative "disease." Rather, we arrive at older age stronger than ever, and various interventions enable us to accommodate a number of chronic conditions at one time, extending the length of time we are able to live with them. This length of time has become significant epidemiologically, sociologically, and economically.

The Second Longevity Revolution

It may be harder to see the second longevity revolution because we are living through it now. This revolution has resulted from our having a better understanding of the impact of lifestyle on survival throughout the lifespan, knowledge that has lengthened life expectancy by an average of 8 years.[6] It can be hard to realize that the sometimes seemingly unremarkable changes that we make are producing a profound change in how long we live. Compared with the larger gains in life expectancy that came from the first longevity revolution, this 8-year increase may seem small. But the increase will undoubtedly continue as we arrive in later life healthier. I was in a unique position to witness these changes in longevity during my decades working with aging adults. The profile of the cohort changed as the years passed.

Since most of us do not even recognize all of the developments that are increasing longevity and the size of the older population, it's time someone wrote about them. Factors range from flu-shot programs to antismoking campaigns, seatbelt laws, and regulations that protect us from industrial dumping and infrastructure accidents. We have come to assume that we have a right to be protected from injury and harm. Societal support for this attitude is evidenced by the enormous increase in civil lawsuits seeking redress from harm caused by unsafe products or practices. Woe is the lot of the corporation that sells defective cars, produces pain medication that causes heart attacks, or fails to clear snowy sidewalks in front of its stores. We no longer tolerate even one death from food poisoning. Our intolerance for risk has reduced the toll taken by defective products to a very low level, especially when compared with where it was in the early 20th century. We now see preventable premature death as something we can and should arm ourselves against. One result of this attitude that is not often noted is the presence of more people who live to be 85 because they have been protected from many kinds of accidents and neglect.

We have filed down the dangerous, sometimes lethal, sharp edges of the built world. Sidewalk cuts and ramps that make it possible to roll a wheelchair or a stroller from one level to the other have become so common that we don't notice them, as have parking spaces for disabled people and easy-grip utensils. State and federal legislation from the 1980s and 1990s made it easier for people with disabilities to use the same facilities as typically developing individuals. The belief that we should accommodate people of every physical capability is as inextricably woven into our cultural fabric as our insistence on the right to enjoy protection from tainted food or an unhealthy environment. By making the world easier to live in, we have made it an easier place for older adults to continue aging, avoid accidents, and engage in activities that keep them physically and mentally healthier. The big square button with the wheelchair icon that opens the automatic door everywhere is pushing up life expectancy whether we realize it or not.

These days, the federal government issues dietary guidance and mandates publication of ingredients on food packaging. Who in 1950 could have imagined that decades later supermarket shoppers would study labels to see whether the frozen waffles contain trans fats or whether the cranberry juice is sweetened with high fructose corn syrup? Diet has become part of the national conversation. We may not always do what's good for us, but we know much more about how to do it. The benefits of exercise have received similar attention, as have the dangers of smoking. A portion of the population is living longer because of this kind of information. The findings of medical research on lifestyle risk factors in whole populations are making contributions to longevity that are comparable to the conquests of infectious diseases in the first half of the 20th century. Improved data are producing masses of health-promoting information. That knowledge has been rapidly translated from medical journals to popular magazines and bestsellers such as Michael Roizen's *Real Age: Are You as Young as You Can Be?* Roizen compiled a list of 129 factors and 74 steps that can help reduce your biological age by up to 20 years.[7] Finding ways to stay healthy and feel younger has become big business, and nothing gets the word out better than big businesses looking for customers. The resulting lifestyle changes lengthen lives, pushing up the trend line for life expectancy. We arrive in old age healthier and therefore keep on getting older.

Advances in medical care are also providing longevity gains beyond the conquering of infectious disease that took place in the early 20th century. Developments in imaging and drug design may have added as many as 3 years to life expectancy. Equally significant has been the development of joint replacement surgery. Rather than ending up in a wheelchair that limits daily activity and breaks down the social network, the older person now benefits from increased mobility and freedom from pain, adding quality to years of life. Pacemakers, defibrillators, and cardiac bypass surgery extend life expectancy in dozens of ways.

Cumulative Advances

All the ways we improve our chances of staying alive, from fire-retardant pajamas to kneeling buses to magnetic resonance imaging, produce large numbers of extra years, but the causes are too many and the progress too multifaceted to take in at a glance. For example, Robert Fogel suggested that the crediting of our increased longevity to modern medicine may be overstated. He argued that, in earlier times, sparse food production and distribution resulted in poor diets and malnutrition, which produced low body weight and stunted height, factors that are predictive not only of vulnerability to infectious disease, but also of chronic conditions in older age. The dramatically increased height and weight of better-nourished World War II veterans compared with Union Army veterans was followed by "a decline of about 35% in the prevalence of chronic disease."[8]

We don't see our own evolution into long lives because the factors that contribute to increased longevity are so many that they are hard to isolate from other dimensions of life. The powerful wind of change in the culture is as invisible as air. Even researchers who study aging do not agree on the nature of this great moment in human history, when so many of us are living so much longer. We don't know if the increase will continue or if we are approaching the limit of how old humans can be. This lack of understanding about the dramatic changing nature of aging has delayed us from seeing it as it really is.

For example, a theorist whose work framed our thinking about the longevity revolution was a Stanford University medical researcher named James Fries, who in 1980 published an influential paper, "Aging, Natural Death, and the Compression of Morbidity" in the *New England Journal of Medicine*. He proposed that the chronic illnesses that affect so many older adults could be staved off until the very end of life so that we live in good health until the very end of the human lifespan, which he projected to be 85 years. In his construction, after that point everything falls apart pretty quickly and we die.

He proposed, in other words, that we would enjoy better health but not longer life. He predicted that "the number of very old persons will not increase, that the average period of diminished physical vigor will decrease, that chronic disease will occupy a small proportion of the typical life span, and that the need for medical care in later life will decrease."[9] Because he didn't know at the moment he was writing that the chronological age of very old people was going to be increasing, he drew the wrong conclusion.

Since the late 20th century, the record clearly shows that older adults are much healthier than they used to be, but contrary to Fries' expectations, they do not die when delayed degenerative diseases finally set in. Apparently, they didn't listen to him! They just keep getting older, even though they are increasingly burdened with their diseases. Fries' misperception had enormous mistaken consequences for age-related policy. Until quite late in the 20th century, the dominant idea was that the time span of chronic conditions would shrink rather than lengthen. This delayed appropriate societal recognition and response to the actual challenge accumulating in our midst.

To recap, for many reasons—from medical advances to societal safety nets—life expectancy has increased overall for most socioeconomic groups, and with it the size of the older population. This is an enormous shift. According to anthropologists, life expectancy probably fluctuated between 20 and 40 years until just a few centuries ago, when it started to climb.[10] That means that for most of human history, old age as we know it now was a rarity. Today, advanced age is normal, and death at younger ages is relatively rare for many demographic groups. That evolution is a change so great that it almost makes us a new species. Surprisingly, we barely feel the change even if we know the facts, and we certainly don't acknowledge its scale and impact. What could possibly be as transforming as the fact that life expectancy has jumped from 47 years to almost 80 years, providing us with the likelihood of 20, 30, or 40 years of life that earlier generations did not have? Perhaps it has been masked by the fact that no dramatic breakthrough announced the longevity revolution. No single discovery led to the longer life we enjoy. It is as if longer life simply materialized around us. Even when we see some of the consequences of the new longevity, we don't recognize the growth of the population of older adults as their cause.

If the increase in longevity had occurred in only half the population so that there was an obvious contrast between one group living longer lives and another dying sooner, it might be easier to see the effects of extended lives.* Several centuries from now, it will look as if someone discovered something in the 20th century that doubled life expectancy. People will wonder then how it felt to live at that amazing moment when life got so much longer, but as we experience it now, it feels like a gradual change.

Another reason we may not readily comprehend the impact of the new longevity is that the difference, first and foremost, is one of quantity. It is not older adults who are the new thing in the world. It's the number of them, a feature that is not immediately evident in the course of a day. Whether we see the change or not, however, our new long lives are bending the world into new shapes.

There has been remarkably little written about the effects of the demographic change. Although there is plenty of discussion of specific issues associated with aging, such as geriatric healthcare or financial planning in retirement, there is very little discussion of what our new long life means in everyday situations or as a big picture. Two years after Fries' article, John Naisbitt's 1982 bestseller *Megatrends: Ten New Directions Transforming our Lives*, listed the forces that would shape the world in the near future. The book said nothing about aging.[11]

We are not looking at the features of society that would show us the revolution because we have not known that we should. We see societal shifts in aging but don't realize how much they owe to increased longevity. I hope the examples that follow, which haven't been collected before as part of an analysis of the changes in aging, will reveal how profoundly increased longevity has transformed our world.

Women's Lives

In 1900, when life expectancy was less than 50 years, a woman would usually marry at a fairly young age and raise children into her middle years. Infant death made it necessary to bear more children

---

*Inner-city minority populations and Native Americans haven't shared the bounty. See: Bharmal, N., Tseng, C.-H., Kaplan, R., Wong, M.D. State-level variations in racial disparities in life expectancy. *Health Services Research.* 2012;47(1, pt. 2), 544–555. https://www.ncbi.nlm.nih.gov/pmc/articles/PMC3393007/.

than we do now, limiting opportunities for women to pursue other activities. If a woman survived childbearing and the infectious diseases that were still a constant threat, her last child might leave the family when she was in her 50s. Her husband would probably work into his 60s and die a few years after retirement, if he retired at all. Robert Fogel noted, "in 1890, nearly everyone died on the job, and if they lived long enough not to die on the job, the average age of retirement was 85."[12] After her husband's death, a woman would typically face a fairly brief widowhood.

A woman born in 1965, on the other hand, if she chose to have children, would expect to have several decades of life after they left the nest. A great difference for these two women separated by half a century was that the first lived in a world in which mortality was a defining condition, common at any age. The other lived in a world in which mortality was pushed almost completely to the end of a long lifespan. We have gone from the early 20th century, when 2 years was the average time spent in retirement, to the early 21st century, when the average woman spends 20.1 years in retirement, and the average man spends 17.1 years.[13] In one century, this is 10 times the years of retirement, and over 40% of her early 1900s life expectancy.

This new expectation of long life is an important reason, not often included among the causes cited in gender studies, that women insisted on joining the workforce in large numbers in the second half of the 20th century. Greater longevity allowed women to seek equality and secure their own destinies by working, not to mention the fact that they needed to sustain themselves for 40 or 50 additional years. The family of a century ago was a unit whose primary purpose was to produce the next generation. Now, with much greater certainty of producing viable offspring who would live into a long adulthood, there are more choices available in other areas of life.

Demography

In addition to their impact on gender roles, changes in life expectancy also play a significant part in demographic shifts that are reshaping the world. It takes 2.1 births per woman to keep a population at a steady level. Demographers call this the *replacement rate*. In the

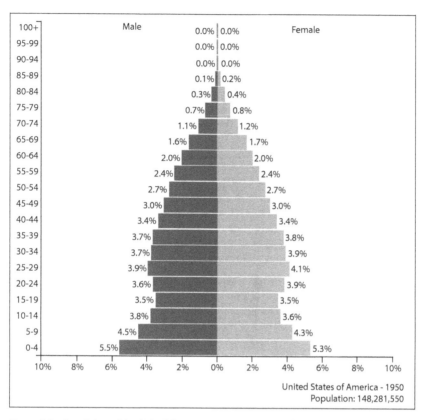

Figure 1.1. Population of the United States in 1950. Source: PopulationPyramid.net. https://creativecommons.org/licenses/by/3.0/igo/legalcode

United States today, as in most developed countries, the birth rate is lower than the replacement rate.[†]

Until recently, a U.S. Census Bureau graphical representation of national population numbers usually looked like a pyramid, with the youngest part of the population as the widest segment at its base and narrowing numbers at each higher age level (see Figure 1.1). At age 85, as I mentioned previously, for every person at the top of the pyramid, there were more than 600 people below. In 2050, there will be just 20

[†] "[I]n 2018 . . . it was estimated that U.S. women would have, on average, 1.73 kids in their lifetimes." [Livingston, G. Is fertility at all-time low? Two of three measures point to yes. Pew Research Center. May 22, 2019. https://pewresearch.org/topic/other-topics/birth-rate-fertility/.]

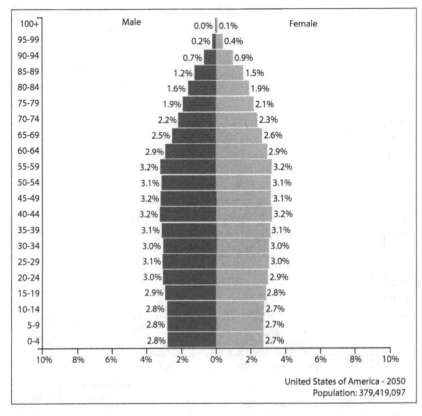

Figure 1.2. Population of the United States projected for 2050. Source: PopulationPyramid.net. https://creativecommons.org/licenses/by/3.0/igo/legalcode

people below for every 85-year-old at the top. The diagram won't be a pyramid, but something closer to an obelisk (see Figure 1.2).

Furthermore, when there were more than 600 people for every person over 85, the financial burden of sustaining the 85-year-old was spread across a broad base. Family units were their own little pyramid schemes, with children providing resources to support their parents. As the population pyramid becomes more columnar, however, broader at the upper reaches of old age and dramatically narrower at the base, the traditional support system goes bust.

The dramatic impact of aging on population pyramids is driving much of the present political turmoil in the Western world. Traditional support for older adults requires the availability of a caregiving younger population of a size that low fertility rates don't sustain.[14] When there are as many 85-year-olds as 8-year-olds, drastically fewer resources exist to support the older group. To keep things running at a steady state, countries whose populations are not replacing themselves have accepted, if not always welcomed, large numbers of immigrants from countries with high unemployment. Underneath the tumultuous political winds regarding immigration is an inexorable need for workers to serve the needs of older adults. The need for workers draws immigrants from Mexico and Latin America and, to a smaller extent, from Asia. The scale of the aging-driven population changes is a major factor in the social tensions at our border entry points.

The aging phenomenon reaches beyond the West and will inform our relationship to our global competitors. An article in *The Lancet*[15] projected that in 2100, China's population will have decreased 48%, from 1.41 billion to 782 million. Japan's population is projected to shrink 59%, from 128 million to 53 million. The consequences of increased longevity and reduced fertility are exaggerated by the one-child policy implemented in China from 1979 to 2013 and by the lack of immigration due to xenophobia in Japan.[16] Education, access to birth control, urbanization, and changing roles for women have created a "demographic momentum."[17] As a result, China and Japan are addressing the dramatic impacts of aging now. They are marshaling technological resources, networks, and robots, giving these countries a head start in the race to capture the lead in a worldwide industry.[18] The U.S. government should secure a share of this enormous developing aging market.

Student Debt

Aging is an unseen, even silent shaper of other seeming unrelated dimensions of life in the United States. Jonathan Zimmerman states that the current $1.7 trillion in outstanding student debt[19] is larger than our collective debt on credit cards.[20] The debt is spread out among 48 million borrowers,[21] almost 20% of Americans over age 18. The precipitous rise of costs burdens families who may defer retirement investments or remortgage their houses. Zimmerman indicates that, "underwritten mainly by private dollars, college is no longer regarded as a public good: it is a personal investment on the part of individuals and their families."[22]

What happened? Why did government funding for higher education sink, leaving the next generation and their families exposed? The short answer is aging. Funding for Medicaid, a program that spends large amounts on older adults, squeezed out state investment in higher education. Peter Orszag, former Director of the Office of Management and Budget, and Thomas Kane, Professor of Education and Economics at Harvard, wrote almost two decades ago that "the expansion in state spending on Medicaid between 1988 and 1998 can explain about 80 percent of the decline in state funding on higher education over the same time period."[23]

Orszag and Kane proceeded to explain that every state dollar allocated to Medicaid has matching federal funding attached. There is no such match for a state's investment in higher education, making the latter less appealing to the state legislature. They foresaw that "projected increases in Medicaid costs over the next several decades thus raise serious questions about the future path of state appropriations for public higher education."[24] Although few today realize the connection between our growing aging cohort and student debt, their projections have held true. Twenty years after Orszag and Kane's study, Temple University Professor Douglas Webber writes that "public welfare spending (primarily Medicaid) . . . account(s) for between 53 percent and 100 percent of the decline in higher-education support."[25]

Healthcare

Aging is also a major underlying cause of the financial crisis in healthcare. With so many more very old adults, there is more need for frailty-related care. Put that increase together with the even more extreme decrease in the prevalence of acute disease and the rise of chronic conditions, and the result is a radically different environment from the one our present healthcare system was built for. This transformation is so central to this discussion that it is the subject of a later chapter.

The changes to longevity and the aging population affect many other elements of society that are not even discussed here. Actuaries need to understand what is happening with life expectancy because insurance companies set rates based on how long buyers of their products will live. Governments need to know trends in longevity because so many social programs, such as housing, healthcare, Social Security, and government pensions, are affected by the length of people's lives. Aging is already 40% of federal spending, and it will be 50% in less than 10 years.[26]

Conclusion

The recent phenomenal increase in our longevity has already made an epochal difference in the way we live as well as our gender roles, generational balance, national borders, education system, retirement support, healthcare expenses, and government spending. Even so, we don't sufficiently appreciate the extent to which aging drives these changes. We don't yet see the increase in longevity for the force it is. We may think of older adults as frail, weak, and powerless, living in an extra stage of life, but they are a growing population that by sheer mass alone tilts everyone younger into a different position in the world. One of the purposes of this book is to bring that fact to everyone's attention. The older adults of the world are an irresistible force and an immovable object.

CHAPTER 2

Where Are the Older Adults?

As discussed, we usually do not perceive the changes in our environment that are lengthening life and the dramatic effects of increased longevity. We are also barely aware of the new character of older adults in our midst. They are a kind of dark matter we can't see among the fixed stars of our outdated mental images of old age. If we look around for what, in loose talk, we call "old people" who fit the outdated stereotype, we will see a few. If we look around instead for "adults over 70," we will find a lot more. In 1950, 70 was old. Now, that's no longer true. So, what does "old" mean today?

New Experiences at Older Ages

A very accomplished, active 89-year-old friend recently had heart bypass surgery, quickly recovered, and told me how astounded he was that he didn't feel as if he was 89. In fact, this is how 89 often feels today. Many older adults are healthy and vigorous, sailing and hiking and dancing at romantic getaways. They are drinking coffee, joking in a noisy supermarket, swimming laps in a pool, or driving home to walk the dog. Many older people are now keenly aware that good physical fitness keeps them safer, more alert, happier, and probably alive longer. They work out; compete in sports; diet; undergo cosmetic surgery; and spend time outdoors jogging, gardening, or golfing.

A small fraction of those who fit our outdated profile of old still exists. We still find elderly women in shawls rocking on their porches, but not as many of them as before. There are some frail women lying in nursing home beds, or what we called fragile old folks leaving church leaning on the arms of their 65-year-old sons and daughters. But these "old" adults are a small percentage of the aging population, and these days they are more likely to be 95 than 75.

People are also stepping out of the stereotypical classification of old by ameliorating the losses that come with aging. Some older persons can diagnose and tune themselves with remarkable acuity. They change their diet, sleeping patterns, as-needed medications, and activity levels at will. They are like the car hobbyist who is so completely familiar with how his 50-year-old car works that he can listen to the most minute creaks and keep it running like new. Their self-repairing maintenance routines lessen the effects of the years. Experienced older adults can combine knowledge, curiosity, and sensitivity to their own bodies and minds to address in minute detail what they need. If it's more effective to live on ground beef than steak, who cares? The object is to stay alive and feel as well as possible. The combination of self-knowledge and self-awareness produces some very old people who are carefully and intricately held together. As old as they may be in years, they may not appear to belong in the group too commonly counted as old.

Some of the interventions introduced recently into the physical world, described previously, have contributed to this new profile of an older adult. We have reduced the effect of some diminished abilities that can come with advanced age by making the built environment more ergonomically friendly to aging gaits and grips. Accommodations for mobility, such as curb cuts and wider doors, have brought many older adults out among us. Medicine relieves the pain and treats the symptoms of some chronic conditions. Joint replacements are a particularly important factor in the changing presentation of those who are old in years but not in appearance or activity. The older person struggling to walk looks older than the same individual taking a stroll after a hip replacement. Many of those with replacement parts will not be perceived as old anymore.

Some older adults are so enmeshed in their age cohort that they don't know they are old. In an airplane 6 miles up, we don't experience the 575–mile-per-hour speed. Relative to our fellow passengers, we are not moving at all. If older adults are more involved with people their own age, they don't feel the wind on their skin as time. The more of their cohort that survives, the more they are buffered from loss. The classic old people of our mind's eye suffered isolation as their contemporaries disappeared. Today's 85-year-old golfer grew up and grew old during the recent lengthening of life expectancy, and this person has a lot more company than his or her grandmother would have had if she had lived to the same age. If enough of us are within reach, we're not old to each other, nor do we seem old to those who watch us enjoying life.

People now pay serious money, if they can, to belong to gyms, buy exercise equipment, and employ personal trainers. A whole industry of books disseminates ways to maximize the body's potential through exercise, food, supplements, rest, and psychology, with specialized programs for all ages. The physically fit white-haired jogger who vigorously circles the block every day does not register as old by former standards. The older gentleman with the knotted biceps at the helm of his sailboat in an ad for an investment management company and the older woman whacking tennis balls in an ad for arthritis medication have no place in our old-fashioned definition of old. They won't be found in rocking chairs. They have disappeared from their porches and gone out into the crowd.

Of course, achieving this energized status requires time, money, and knowledge of what needs to be done, so not all older adults can reach such levels. Perhaps some of the changes in the delivery system suggested later in this book can alleviate the disparities caused by socio-economic status and make the new version of being old more widely available.

Misperceptions

I am part of the generation called the Baby Boomers, born between 1944 and 1964. What age looked like to us when we were children forming our images of older adults in the 1950s and 1960s is embedded in our memories. Back then we encountered most older people as worn down and financially strapped. They would pass over a line that separated them from the "not old." We often retain those early ideas about people who have reached certain chronological age markers. The residual images of the last years of life that were baked into us in our childhoods may result in unnecessary fear and even prejudice against and rejection of older adults.

The confused old person, one of the standard types we used to know, was actually misclassified. Instead of dismissing the individual as "senile," we now recognize him or her as having dementia, a disease that is not an inevitable consequence of normal aging. Those with dementia have moved out of the set labeled "older adults" and into a set identified as "people with medical conditions."

In similar fashion, until late in the 20th century, depression in an older adult was often assumed to be a normal consequence of aging. It seemed reasonable that someone would be depressed when he or she had lost so much. But depression, which occurs in all stages of life, can often be treated as successfully in the old as in the young. The grieving uncle in the corner at the family gathering does not need to languish with no interventions. When his mood improves, he will seem and feel less old. We can often fine-tune older adults' behavior to prevent or rescue them from the emotional decrepitude that can develop from the losses associated with old age. Even in the arena of physical intimacy, pharmaceuticals have restored vigor to men who believed their sex lives were over.

It was also true throughout much of the 20th century that even though most older adults were poor, they might be fortunate enough to be living on the kindness of family, for which they may have been humbly appreciative. Social welfare programs, the modernization of pensions, and in some cases the appreciation of assets have combined to raise some older people to a level of at least moderate independent comfort. In recent economic busts, a portion of older adults was actually hurt less because their houses were paid for and they had incomes from defined benefit plans. Keep in mind, however, that while many people have sufficient resources to be comfortable during their relatively healthy retirement years, they are almost completely unprepared financially for profound frailty.

New Knowledge and a New World for Older Adults

Social gerontologists study older adults to learn how they experience different situations. The work of these researchers has updated the picture of life in older age. Understanding the disorientation and concomitant destabilizing effects that come from being trundled from one strange place (a hospital) to another (a rehab setting), for example, has led to devising protocols and interventions that mitigate confusion and distress. There is now a new cohort of psychologists, social workers, caseworkers, and care team leaders who evaluate older adults. The interventions that work are often ones that were developed specifically for gerontological needs. Where an older person's poor fit with an unyielding environment might once have begun to reduce his or her competence, now social services can intervene.

As described previously, our world is different from the way it was during all the past millennia of humankind because so many people now live to very old age. At the nursing home where I worked for 30 years, it was sometimes possible to see brief flickers of astonishment and incomprehension in the oldest residents. Very old women born around 1900, when life expectancy was low, had formed their impressions of life according to the norms of their time. They had grown up in a world in which dying in one's 60s was seen as normal rather than as dying young. They had lived through the demographic transition from the time when the average length of life was 47 years to the era when it had stretched to 80 and beyond.

When members of the World War II (WWII) generation were 30 years of age, 577,000 Americans were over 85. When they turned 60, the over-85 cohort had increased to 2.2 million. While the parents of the WWII generation had been isolated castaways blown onto an unknown planet of long life, they themselves had become numerous enough to colonize it. Now *their* children, the Baby Boom generation, are fully established on that planet. In 2050, when all the Boomers are over 85, the Census Bureau estimates that there will be 19 million of them. I had a front-seat view of this transition unfolding while working in a nursing home in the 1980s. But to many who do not have this vantage point, it isn't so easy to see the new situation of older adults, even though there are now so many more of them and they are changing our world.

The WWII generation—the parents of the Baby Boomers—were often silent about their own experiences of getting older, leaving their offspring with no clear picture of the experience. They had endured much more difficult economic times and had much lower levels of education. There must have been little residual energy for talking about quality of life. It has only been during the Boomers' lifetimes that interest in how people think and express themselves about their personal experiences has grown to be a significant part of the culture. Although there were merely a few decades between many in the WWII and Boomer generations, there was a gap in how each experienced the world, and especially in how each communicated about these experiences. Because their parents rarely discussed what it was like to be 70, Boomers could only imagine what the experience was like. They are now coming to realize that their experience may be very different from what their parents led them to expect. The biggest surprise for many comes from recognizing the continuing vibrancy of their minds. It had not occurred to them that their own personal experience in older age would actually be a new age of living that they had not anticipated, filled with interesting activities, new knowledge, and fulfilling relationships.

Conclusion

We Boomers will probably be the last generation to see aging in the old-fashioned way. We are beginning to reach the age our grandparents were when we were children, and we are not behaving as they did. The understanding of old age that children are acquiring in the 21st century is also new. They didn't grow up visiting grandparents and great-grandparents who presented in the old stereotypes. If all members of today's over-65 population wore neon green safety vests with the word "OLD" in large letters on the backs, they would be easy to perceive. Instead, whether we see them or not depends on what we're looking for. And what we're looking for probably depends on our own age. There is little literature that helps to explore today's very different nature of this period of older adulthood. Boomers will have to discover and map it for themselves, and for their sons and daughters.

CHAPTER 3

Aging Care in the Present

A Holdover from the Industrial Age

I hope it is clear from the preceding chapters that we have an explosion of individuals whose presence is having an enormous influence on our society, even though we are not always aware of their impact. This became clear to me as I watched the cohort of old people change. I also realized that we need to find new and better ways of providing older adults with safety, care, and activity. Because the modern era enables so many to live long enough to accumulate chronic conditions, most of the adults that I have been describing are going to need interventions, even though they may need them much later than has been the case in previous generations. Since there are so many more of them, the challenge will be enormous. As I will describe in Chapter 6, I believe that we are going to achieve those goals by using the technology of the modern Digital Age instead of Industrial Age models. The result will be a less costly and happier existence for our oldest generation.

The Old Way

In order to understand how this transformation in the lives of older adults is going to happen, let's recall what their lives have been like for the last 100 years or so. The traditional model that I am about to describe has begun to change here and there but is still the dominant one. It no longer fits the new circumstances stemming from the much greater numbers of older people, their new longevity, and their many additional years of health and well-being. The gap between what has actually already changed in the aging population and our lagging understanding of and response to it is creating unnecessary difficulties. Older adults, with their larger numbers and longer lives, need accommodations from society right now. They are suffering because of our inaction. Very frail older adults in particular have less power to control their circumstances and have to endure the most dire consequences of living in a world that has not caught up with changed times. If we continue to create miserable and unsuitable living conditions for older adults because we cannot yet see the approaches that would work better, we are letting our oldest generation live and die with suffering that could be avoided.

Below is a description of the typical experience of aging as it too often evolves even up through the early 21st century, when an older person and a caregiving daughter attempt to navigate the Industrial Age patterns of aging care in the United States. I have witnessed many iterations of this story. Although it may now happen when the mother turns 90 rather than 75, its basic outline has not changed.

One Mom's Story

After many years of a healthy and vigorous life, small things that are slightly askew in Mom's behavior become more noticeable and slowly create the recognition that Mom isn't just being difficult or stubbornly forgetful; she actually needs more help. The routines that Mom has developed to fill in for the changes she is sensing start to become less adequate. Gradually, the daughter takes on Mom's tasks for her, managing her bank account, her car, her various appointments, and her bills, trying not to hurt Mom's pride or arouse her anger.

Then comes the twilight. With greater age comes a cascade of challenges, which family members work to address but never overcome completely. Even when a new adjustment helps, it doesn't hold for long because Mom continues to change. Problems interact with each other, making each change, move, or interaction a gamble, for there are too many unknowns that need to enter into the calculation. One issue sets off another in a never-ending swirl. Aides visit, but as Mom's needs multiply, it becomes more and more difficult to have help at the ready at the exact moment the need arises. Some days proceed smoothly; some don't. Professional advice and services come and go. All approaches are so specialized that, even when they have merit in themselves, it is not worthwhile to try to integrate them into the flow of interventions. Surrounded by specialists, the daughter is alone.

As Mom's patterns fall away, they cease to be patterns at all. Over time, lack of judgment morphs into confusion and incoherence—at least nothing that is coherent to the daughter. Mom's lucidity does reappear intermittently. The daughter, frustrated, looks in vain for the logic to explain the pattern of when and why her mother reappears.

The number of translations and transformations–physical, cognitive, financial, emotional–don't evolve easily or flow smoothly. The interrelated issues never stop moving and clashing. One problem sets up another in a never-ending, tightening swirl. The daughter adjusts Mom's environment and then adjusts it again, first at her apartment, then at her assisted-living suite. Even in those environments, the daughter continues to supplement and negotiate as Mom's constantly changing conditions move her in and out of an appropriate fit within each facility's set program. With each move, how will Mom respond? Will the new setting be better? Can she, or we, afford it?

The daughter watches as the pieces of the mother she knew disappear in front of her eyes. She pumps out energy, making choices and negotiating with Mom. Hypervigilance becomes habitual. It feels as if there is no way out. The daughter endures waves of panic, relief, and anger. She realizes that Mom's care has taken over her own life, pushing other relationships to the periphery. Mom is not even aware or appreciative of her efforts, which leads to welling resentment. No one is okay.

The Old Solution

One frequent answer to the dilemma of how to care for an aging person when the family can no longer do so has been the traditional nursing home. When I started working in aging care in the early 1980s, nursing homes mimicked the floor plans of hotels or hospitals. The basic model had bedrooms lining long corridors. This worked well enough for the relatively well 75- to 80-year-olds who lived in them at the time and whose primary need was for shelter and safety. Nursing homes were more like orphanages for older adults than healthcare facilities, more like dormitories than hospitals. Residents would get up in the morning and use the bathrooms, dress, walk down the corridor to the elevator, and ride downstairs for dining, therapy, and socializing on the ground floor.

In the late 20th and early 21st centuries, nursing home populations grew older as overall longevity increased. By 2000, the nursing home resident was likely to be an 85- to 95-year-old with very limited abilities. These new "old folks" can no longer dress themselves and make their way downstairs for meals and activities. They cannot communicate directly. They need special food and specialized equipment. Dealing with the body's natural outputs is a challenge. The residents in the mid-20th century were comparatively capable, but the residents of the early 2000s cannot get down the corridor to the elevators on their own. The staff is too busy to transport them in good time for meals and activities. When residents do get downstairs, they need to be taken to the bathroom frequently. With their cognitive, hearing, and vision losses, they cannot socialize easily. Yet the typical nursing home hasn't changed its arrangement to match the new profile of the typical resident. It is not a happy situation.

As a result of these mismatches between person and environment, residents usually stop coming downstairs. They live along their corridors, in environments that have little air circulation and outside light and no spaces to gather in groups. Most nursing homes were built years ago to accommodate dramatically fewer wheelchairs because so many more people died at earlier ages. The bathrooms adjacent to the rooms aren't large enough for safe transfers from wheelchair to toilet. In order to get to the toilet safely, residents in wheelchairs have to use the larger public bathrooms. The inhabitants of this outdated living arrangement sit queued up in the corridor waiting for the toilet, hoping not to have an accident, trying to synchronize bowel or bladder needs to the progress of the line.

There is no place to put the supplies and equipment necessary for this older and more frail population, so carts of clean and dirty linen, food, and dirty dishes are also lined up in the corridors. Residents, equipment, and supplies are all batch processed. There is no individualization, much less systems that provide people with coffee when they want it or let them enjoy individual activities or private time according to their own wishes. The result enervates and deflates all the participants and repels outsiders. The smell of urine and feces that spreads through the environment makes the home feel dirty. Even if the physical environment is hygienically clean, with pervasive incontinence and the lack of air flow, it smells like human waste.

The result is dehumanizing for the residents. After 90 years of living, a slow decline or a sudden accident rips an older adult out of the environment shaped around his or her history and thrusts the person into a stark, remote environment that doesn't recognize his or her individuality. Familiar routines are simply no longer available. The older person is profoundly distressed at having been pulled out of his or her life and is now completely dependent on caregivers. Frustration turns to anger and then turns inward to depression.

The sights, sounds, and smells I have just described were the only world we knew in the mid-20th century, and it continues, substantially unchanged, today. The system is clearly not providing the kind of care we want for our relatives. It is a grim and degraded existence but, unless an exhausted son or daughter cares for the profoundly frail adult at home, we have not produced another way.

New Approaches

The first step in my own journey of trying to solve problems for older adults started in the 1980s when I went to work in a nursing home like the one described previously, where frail old men and women were doing "hard time." With a small and dedicated team of forward thinkers, including an environmental psychologist, an architect, and some receptive community members, we endeavored to re-create the model of the nursing home to provide safety and care to very old fragile adults while still preserving their individuality, dignity, and freedom despite their reduced capabilities. Even though our project, which I will describe in Chapter 4, was a success—in fact, a national award–winning success—it wasn't the end of the story. What we thought was a model was really a stage in a far longer-range project. In the beginning, we started by asking how we could improve the lives of the older people we were caring for. A few decades later, we made our way to another question: Wouldn't it be better to retain the very old in the communities where the rest of us live? That is where my story will lead.

Who was I to believe that I could solve so large a problem? In my early 30s, after obtaining a law degree and serving a brief stint in the family apparel business, I realized I needed an occupation in which to lose myself. Someone a generation older than I, who was an executive in the field of aging, described caring for the aging to me and opened a new world. The field involved caring for vulnerable, needy people, and that appealed to my idealism. I went back to school to study applied gerontology in a program at North Texas State University (now the University of North Texas) in Denton. I served three internships in different long-term care facilities, read everything I could find about aging and management, and eventually found a job in Buffalo, New York.

I was looking for meaningful work and stimulation. Care for older people was clearly in need of a radical remaking. I knew I was walking into territory where everything was in motion, but in my early years in the field, I didn't understand that aging was profoundly remaking the world. The changes from the longevity revolution were still very new in the 1980s, and no one was noticing them yet. Now I can see that what was, and still is, happening with aging is as life changing and pervasive as the arrival of the computer chip. That's a big part of my message in this book.

The advent of the Digital Age has been the subject of far more discussion and writing than has been the arrival of a massive cohort of older adults. The disparity in interest is noteworthy. Of course, some issues in aging get discussed, such as how to reduce expenses in retirement or safeguard the kitchens of our aging parents, probably because the Baby Boomer generation is now caring for mothers and fathers, and because the first of the Boomers are themselves entering older age. We are also more interested in aging because it looks like, as a society, we won't have the money to pay for its care. But we tend to talk about particular aging issues as they pop up. We don't see them against a background; we don't fit them into a comprehensive understanding.

Conclusion

From the outset, I sensed I was living through a period that separated an old world from a new one, even if I didn't understand it right away. As I will describe, I built a large, award-winning healthcare system that reconfigured how to deliver care for our frail older population. My career focused on the practical management of care for frail older adults. In the process I acquired a horizon-to-horizon view of aging. What I think about older age, healthcare, architecture, management theory, policy, and the economics of care comes from decades of actually delivering it. In the pages that follow, I will describe the successes and failures of our enterprise and our innovations, as well as explore why they turned out to be only steps along the way to a more profound reconfiguration of attitudes toward and treatment of aging.

CHAPTER 4

Attempting to Address the Problem

The New Home

As I have described, when I entered the field of aging in the 1980s, all the consequences of increased longevity and the larger numbers of older adults were just beginning to make themselves felt, albeit often unacknowledged. Longer life expectancy was quietly producing a new kind of old age. The increase in the number of people living much longer was often not recognized, in part because so many of them were aging so well. No preparation was being made for the upcoming deluge of their frail years, when their housing needs and healthcare would require support. Unfortunately, the almost exclusive venue for addressing frailty continued to be the nation's nursing home industry.

Finding the Team

I had the good fortune of working for an enlightened board of directors when I moved up to the job of director for an old inner-city nursing home a few months after coming to Buffalo in 1984. I soon realized that the community's state-of-the-art structure, built 10 years before with all good intentions, was based on an outdated Industrial Age model that did not give the residents the quality of life they deserved. When the board asked me to assess the future of the home, I responded that I believed it was serving the wrong people with the wrong programs in the wrong place. I assumed they would shake my hand and send me on my way for my impertinence. To my surprise, they handed me the opportunity to sell the old building and construct a New Home.

I hired Lorraine Hiatt, a young environmental gerontologist specializing in aging, who was already well known for her ideas about how to make environments work better for people in nursing homes. With her as my guide and collaborator, I set out to find the best nursing home model in the United States. After many site visits and much conversation, we realized that all the nursing homes we saw were still anchored, as ours was, in an earlier era. They were not designed to respond to the needs of current residents or the new factors in aging outlined in the previous chapters of this book. The buildings we visited were environments for frail older adults that were more hostile than helpful. Dark, warm, stuffy rooms provided ideal conditions for developing pressure ulcers on sedentary residents. Windowless, uncarpeted, cluttered corridors made falls more likely. Warrens of hallways and rooms with little visual access to the outdoors were particularly disorienting for people in the twilight zones of memory and cognitive decline, producing depression in many.

Despite all the funding and building and regulating of long-term care facilities that had started when states and the federal government got involved in care of the aged in the 1950s and 1960s, the actual facilities themselves had not changed much. Buildings had gotten bigger and shinier and fire safety had improved. But in those years almost all the energy in aging care went into increasing capacity and efficiency. The baseline purpose of aging care facilities was to keep older adults alive and safe. More capacity meant more old people could be accommodated. Quality of life was not very high on the list of priorities. There was no thought of an alternative to the traditional basic model of batch-processing residents assembly-line style.

Our explorations and our experience in our own nursing home in Buffalo gave us a pretty good understanding of why the current model wasn't working for our residents, but we had no idea what alternative system would work. We realized that we needed a place that would not only provide shelter, food, and waste disposal, but also address the real challenges of living and delivering care in a nursing home.

We looked for an architect who could understand both the knowledge provided by the environmental psychologist and the experience we had accumulated working in nursing homes and studying them. We found a small architectural firm that understood that the real clients for the project were the residents and the staff of the New Home, not the board of directors or the donors. The principal architect for our project was the late Zachary Rosenfield. His group turned out to be the right choice for us, but we were taking a gamble when we made it. I had to persuade my board to choose a firm based on how well its staff understood the life of a nursing home resident and the rhythms of the systems surrounding the resident, rather than how attractive the building might seem to outsiders. That may now appear to be an obvious approach but, at the time, thinking about the problem from that angle didn't come naturally to any of us.

Design of the New Home

We started the design process by trying to describe the end result: What did we want the building to do? It was clear that our residents could not get to distant services easily, so we determined that services should come to them. We wanted privacy for them, which meant that the building needed private rooms with accessible private toilets. We wanted a dignified way for the residents to bathe and we wanted them to have visual access to the outside. We wanted to eliminate unpleasant odors and to have convenient but unobtrusive places for equipment. Finally, we wanted our nurse's aides, who are the frontline workforce in a nursing home, to have the means to take care of residents flexibly, responding to individual needs rather than following the assembly-line service delivery that was pervasive in all the nursing homes we knew.

We put the frail older men and women at the center of every discussion, presentation, paper, and whiteboard diagram when we planned the new place. We also started with a belief that the physical environment shaped the nature of the existence of these people. In fact, we later realized that we could trace many of our eventual difficulties in adjusting to the New Home to the moments in the planning when we had lost our focus on the older adults.

What were the needs of frail older residents that we believed we could address through architecture? There were three. The first was privacy: individual space for one's most intimate moments. With great age, strength diminishes, and the world shrinks. As the process of answering bodily needs becomes more complex, dignity is ever more precious and precarious. Sexuality evolves, but it doesn't depart. The loss of privacy when the personal realm is reduced to a bed in a room shared with another can dampen the pleasure of life. A semiprivate room with two beds is not really private at all. For most people, to be thrust into semiprivate space demeans the person in ways that are deeply injurious. Sharing a bathroom is particularly worrisome. One person in the bathroom leaves the other in jeopardy of losing control of his or her bodily functions. So we built only private rooms in the New Home.

After privacy, the second need we addressed was semipublic space, like a front porch on a house might provide. Such a space beckons people out of their private realms to watch the world, perhaps to exchange a word with a passerby. In the world of the nursing home, if that space is comfortable and easily accessible, it can expand the range of the hesitant resident. Worry about bowels and bladder or the need for help can often hold the frail old person back as his or her internal signals and control can become undependable. To have a public accident is an insult to the self. Every step away from the bathroom is fraught with risk. So, the semipublic space must not be far from the private bathroom and must also allow the nurse's aide to remain close at hand. The space should be large enough to hold opportunities for socializing and small activities but not so large that it becomes too noisy and confusing. The benefit of such space in a nursing home is the preservation of the social self.

Third, frail old residents need access to some amount of public space. Without it, people can lose their public personae. Anticipating how others will view one and sprucing up to be seen are important. Retaining an amount of public posture extends the sense of self.

The real challenge in designing the New Home was to find the proper scale and relationship among these three types of space, keeping the older adult's emotional, physical, and psychological needs at the center of the design. Physical space is always precious and finite in a building. We were developing something that had to work financially as well, so that we could pay for it going forward and it could be a practical model to be replicated.

The architect listened to all our dreams, then went away to work with his staff. When he came back, he rolled out the plan on my desk. At first, I couldn't comprehend it. Very gradually, I began to understand his new design/concept—we didn't even know what to call it—and the new delivery system that was an integral part of the plan. Rather than lined up along hallways, the residents' rooms were arranged in small groups of seven or eight around a living room, with sets of four of these small groups gathered around a semipublic space that included a small living room. A dining area for 30 residents was nearby, and there was no large, centralized dining in the building. The large public area was situated outside the private and semiprivate spaces, providing visitors a comfortable, noninvasive environment and an accessible public arena where residents could "go to town." We came to call the basic seven- or eight-room unit in the New Home a "cluster." The new system of delivering care was called "cluster management." When I first absorbed Zach's plan in 1988, I didn't realize that it would take almost 10 years (including 5 years after we moved into the new facility) for everyone else—staff, regulators, other providers, residents, families, and the community—to metabolize these unfamiliar ideas for both architecture and delivery of care.

What we did in the New Home that departed from the standard care model was to change its architecture, which led to changes in how we delivered care, and that, in turn, released our residents from an oppressive regime that had been the best we could do for them up to that time.

Educating the Caregivers

Zach Rosenfield's design for a facility arranged into small clusters of private rooms broke the nursing home away from the assembly-line paradigm. Once understood, it seemed obviously preferable to the old setup of long corridors and batch-processed delivery. But what would it take to change the delivery of care as radically as the design of the building required? How could we translate a set of ideas into actual better living for the residents of our ideal home? We wanted our frontline staff, who worked directly with our residents, dressed them, took them to the toilet, fed them, talked to them, and shared their environment, to come to see their work not as the set of ordered tasks to which they were accustomed, but as a nuanced mosaic of responses to the needs of individuals. Our guiding objective was to integrate quality of *care* and quality of *life* in the new building. The former calls for efficiency, safety, and appropriateness; the latter is a state of emotional well-being. We had to figure out how to balance them properly in a decentralized delivery model. We needed to understand the work of caring for the residents in a completely new way, and then to rebuild its routines.

We approached the challenge in several ways. We engaged facilitators from the Creative Problem Solving Institute, then based at SUNY Buffalo State College, to lead our management team through thinking about the new cluster management approach to care that we were inventing, which the new building was designed to support. Their process brought together on a weekly basis the 20 staff members who actually operated the facility to articulate the problems and benefits that the new design would present and to brainstorm solutions when necessary. The results of the process were incorporated into both the physical design and the new management system.

I also asked our management team to read *The Machine That Changed the World: The Story of Lean Production* by Womack, Jones, and Roos, which had just been published.[27] It described how Henry Ford invented the assembly line, with interchangeable parts and interchangeable workers, in order to produce a complex product. Ford broke down the work into a series of small operations, such as attaching a wheel or screwing on a door, so a laborer could learn the technique in a matter of minutes and then repeat it all day. An engineer would lay out a line so that hundreds of discrete, relatively simple and monotonous programmed tasks would produce, almost miraculously, a highly complex product. Only the one at the top who understood the entire system could think through the cascade of changes necessary to accommodate a refinement to the assembly line. Over time, as the book describes, the foundations of this system changed. Workers' costs, with unionization, benefits, and government protections, rose dramatically. Further, the assembly-line model that had modernized and urbanized the United States was producing boredom and anger in the workers. Eventually, as a result of inflexibility and dissatisfaction, 30%–50% of cars coming off the assembly line had to be sent back because of quality deficiencies. One response to the declining atmosphere was what has come to be called lean production, in which small-scale teams on the shop floor replace the assembly line. Workers are given access to more information and are retrained to perform multiple operations and charged with the authority to suggest and implement improvements in work methods.

A few chapters into reading this book, our nursing home management team wanted to know why we were reading about automobile plants. My answer was that if we changed "assembly-line worker" to "nurse's aide," the book was about us. In the following 2 years, we created our own lean production, introducing decentralization of food production, activities, bathing, laundry, and supervision. We made hundreds of small-scale course corrections and additions to the new model as we built it.

Struggles and Frustrations

Today, all of this seems agreeably progressive, easy to understand and support. Back then, the work had none of that warm feeling. We were still working in the old corridor-based nursing home as we planned our future systems and as the actual new building rose. Each worker in the nursing home was being asked to imagine changes to long-standing work routines and traditional relationships in a not-yet-existing environment that would theoretically support the new routines, roles, and behaviors we were creating.

We whipped ourselves into a high state of belief in our new model; we reified it in all our daily and weekly problem-solving and decision-making sessions. We did our best to make the new model real, and we learned to make decisions that were consistent with it. We quietly and slowly gave new shape and structure to the organization and to our own thinking. Paradoxically, this increased frustration. The existing building felt more and more like a heavy shroud as we continued to work in it, depriving residents and staff alike of dignity, flexibility, and quality of life. There were tears and anger. Some staff resigned because the proposed changes made them too uncomfortable or seemed wrongheaded.

Our traditional authority-based management style was suddenly challenged and supplanted by a more engaged and democratic one. I had assumed that, as innovative planners, the designers and management team would be received as liberators; that when we struck off their shackles, the staff would embrace individual responsibility as more personally fulfilling. I was stunned by how wrong I was. It never crossed my mind the staff wouldn't love the changes. But work in the traditional nursing home is organized in departmental hierarchies. Many of our long-time staffers had climbed the chain of command. Supervisors were accustomed to making all the decisions. Departments tended to compete with one another for resources and attention, and the competition had become a defining factor in the organizational culture. The concerns of residents and their families had become secondary to department fealty in order to protect staff members' jobs by focusing on protecting each department's responsibilities and prerogatives. So when we introduced new expectations for decision-making at lower levels, for taking individual responsibility, and for accepting the consequences of one's own decisions rather than simply following direction from supervisors, the response was not universally positive. It took thousands of small steps over a long time to develop a more nimble, change-oriented culture, one in which the staff searches for solutions to problems and where continuous improvement is seen as gratifying. Our old systems and behaviors were so ingrained that even extremely capable managers could not always change their fundamental mindsets in the way that was necessary. It took years to develop a responsive, individualized approach to resident needs.

Impact of the New Home

After 6 years of long, laborious planning for the evolution from the old style to the new, we were ready to inhabit the new building. Our great fear was that when we moved 166 residents and 120 staff to an environment that had never been tried before, we would crash. We couldn't afford to let anything go wrong. We started taking staff on trial runs to the new facility. We asked them to imagine doing tasks in the new space, the way athletes visualize perfect routines; we had them talk and walk through their anticipated new daily activities of getting the resident in and out of the bathroom, to the dining table, ready for bed.

The day arrived on August 15, 1993, 5 years after our board of directors had approved the design and 9 years after we began our strategic planning process. Our residents ate breakfast in the old world. All day, buses, cars, vans, and ambulances ferried frail older adults away from the spaces they knew. At the end of the day, we served dinner in the new world. By 9 p.m., everyone was settled in bed, and the new facility was at rest. A new era had begun.

It would be difficult to overestimate the effect of the New Home on our residents' lives. At first, it was nearly incomprehensible. The sights, sounds, and smells of the old place had been so overwhelming we had not imagined they wouldn't come with us. In anticipation of the move, we had examined and analyzed, and either kept, eliminated, or reformatted each component of traditional nursing home life. There were no queues in the New Home. Residents could orient themselves visually to the outside world and could function on their own individual rhythms. Privacy was restored to private tasks; there was minimal traveling for basic human functions. It was quiet. The cumulative effect of the hundreds of adjustments and innovations we had worked through individually was hard to grasp.

The way we learned to handle the laundry is an illustrative example of how we developed new models. When I first arrived at the old nursing home in 1984, families would frequently complain that someone else was wearing Mom's dress. I discovered that the staff would drop all the residents' clean clothes in a single pile in the corridor when they received it from the central laundry each morning. Nurse's aides would rummage through the pile to find clothing to dress their charges. I was appalled, and as I begin to evaluate the problem, I found that often the clothes weren't marked with residents' names and that, even if the items were labeled, many aides couldn't read. Dirty laundry was sent down the laundry chute with the dirty diapers. Everything was batch processed at a single location, where there was no way to tell what garment belonged in what unit, much less to which resident.

The nurse's aides' desperation to get their residents dressed before breakfast not infrequently led to skirmishing for clothing. So, aides would hoard clean clothing in drawers and closets. It was a free-for-all. Because management had not designed an integrated system, the nurse's aides had no other choice but to create their own. Each player did the best he or she could, battling for his or her immediate interests. In the new building, we created a system that made everyone happier. We decentralized laundry by putting a washer and dryer in each small cluster of rooms. An aide would take a resident's dirty laundry from the resident's room and return it 2 hours later.

We realized that many of the behaviors residents had displayed when they were living in the chaotic visual and auditory environment of the old building and had lost their possessions and dignity were not the inevitable results of aging at all. Our residents became calmer and more inclined to engage with one another and with the activities around them. An inappropriate environment had exacerbated their former distress and anxiety. The old building had created one kind of resident, and the new building revealed another, one that seemed to be much more like you and me. Individual needs were now attended to. The flurry and stress of the earlier atmosphere that had compounded the experience of loss and displacement was reduced. Residents were cleaner and better dressed, and it was easier for visitors to spend time with them.

In *Smart World*, Richard Ogle explained that this is how we create and re-create the world to serve us.[28] He said, "we do not rely solely on our mind's internal resources" but we create spaces that think for us. "We live in a smart world."[29] The appropriate height of a chair or lighting in a hallway extends our intelligence, enabling us to reserve our mind's energies for other tasks. In this sense, our environments rob or enhance our physical and cognitive energies. We tried to apply this kind of principle to the environment of the New Home.

Long-Term Picture

In the earliest years of planning and executing the new model, we were exuberant. Looking back, I believe we thought we could remake not just the experience, but the participants as well. We knew the old approach to care had often masked residents' residual competencies. We also believed that the staff's inherent warmth, energy, and engagement were squelched by the industrial-style regime they had to follow, and that these qualities would quickly emerge in our new environment. While much of our theory turned out to be true, the reality, of course, was much more complex.

We believed that the residents and the nursing assistants complemented one another and that the new system would evoke an entirely new culture. What I now understand is that our experience was more like peeling an onion. The new building offered enormous advantages for both residents and care aides. Life and work were easier. But we over-anticipated the goodwill and engagement of many of the "newly freed" staff. Some staff, given new tools and freedoms, rose to wonderful heights, but the new building and our preconceived notions still masked some of the gaps in care. At first, we relaxed our supervisory and management responsibilities. Then, when some staff did not rise to the opportunity, we tried to return to parts of the more traditional command and control systems, but the decentralized building and our entire advance staff training pushed back against this. We learned, carefully and persistently, to put together systems that took both old and new factors into account. It required a long-term effort of constantly analyzing what could be delegated and to whom. Much of what we believed would come to pass actually did, but only after years of grinding hard work, feeling our way toward new approaches to managing and measuring.

Conclusion

In 1994, early in this journey toward a better model of care delivery, we received the National Peter F. Drucker Award for Innovation in Nonprofit Management, the first time a healthcare organization was so honored. I would say we eventually earned the award, but not until another 10 years of hard work and problem solving had passed.

Even when the New Home was finally running smoothly, I still didn't know that we hadn't arrived; we had simply stopped to refit and resupply along the way in a journey that was just beginning. For all our successes, it turned out the journey had more distance to travel. We slowly began to realize that this wasn't the full picture of where we needed to go.

CHAPTER 5

Dealing with Government Bureaucracy

In previous chapters, I have tried to explain the changes that are taking place in the world of aging as well as the need to respond to an enormous population of older adults who will eventually accumulate a variety of frail conditions after having been healthy for longer than has been possible before. The New Home that we built in Buffalo was an attempt to find a solution to the problem by designing a place where older men and women in need of care could live with dignity. It was a success in itself but, as I will explain further in later chapters, this one model will not solve the problem of caring for the size of the coming generations. There will be too many older people to accommodate in such facilities at an attainable cost. We must search for another answer. Along the way to the New Home, we had to overcome some serious roadblocks, which still exist elsewhere. Our experience in dealing with the most difficult of these obstacles, as I will describe in this chapter and the next, will be useful to know about as we and others try to make more changes in the care system for our aging population. Similar difficulties will undoubtedly reappear and need to be dealt with as society moves forward to solutions beyond the New Home.

The layers of government bureaucracy that we constantly encountered created a serious obstacle as we worked to change the paradigm of nursing home care. Not surprisingly, the government does not spend hundreds of billions of dollars without rules and regulations governing how the funds are used. The government programs that cover the cost of custodial care for people are concerned with what residents eat, who dispenses their medication, the incidence of pressure ulcers, and many other particulars. For example, the Federal HUD 202 program subsidizes housing for low-income older adults. It is concerned with the number and size of the rooms and with the kinds of services that must be offered. All this supervision ensures that the program recipients get what the program is designed to provide. State and federal departments regulate everything having to do with government spending in nursing homes such as wheelchair design, institutional meals, qualifications for caregivers, nutritional standards, doorway widths, bathroom layouts, and much more.

This governmental bureaucracy for the care of older people was built to assure safety and fairness, but it makes innovation difficult. The system is a product of the Industrial Age model for aging care, concentrating everything in one place. My New Home, despite its early success, was still conceived on the model of providing care in a single location. Each component of care in the location is based on an Industrial Age linear process. Each component stands alone and the regulations do not allow different institutions and programs to consider interactions between the components. I will describe in a later chapter why this heavily regulated area has resisted technological change, unlike most other commercial sectors in the United States, and is therefore much more difficult to adjust when circumstances change. So, to put the present situation in a nutshell: Our outmoded and costly systems for aging care are almost impossible to change because of the regulations that have grown around them.

Role of the State Government

I remember vividly my first trip to the New York State capital in Albany to seek backing for our new type of nursing home when it was in the planning stages in Buffalo. The monumental scale of Empire State Plaza, home of the New York State Department of Health, stunned me. The closer I approached the department's office tower, the more insignificant my ideas seemed to be. Inside were the endless offices of a highly bureaucratized state healthcare delivery system, the largest in the nation. Its denizens would decide the fate of our project. Environmental gerontologist Lorraine Hiatt, architect Zachary Rosenfield, and I made a series of treks to the state Department of Health. As we went from bureau to bureau, racing deadlines, filing forms, and laying out our wares, I began to perceive a distinctive organizational culture. Its bestriding presence was the spirit of the late, almost mythical David Axelrod, Commissioner of the New York State Department of Health from 1979 to 1991. He died before

I made my first trip to Albany, but the department's leaders still held him in personal and professional awe.

The health department's role in New York State's healthcare system is still deeply informed by the early years of the 20th century, when it was created. New York was then dominated by industry, and people were flocking to cities for work. Packed tenements had only primitive public hygiene. Despite rapidly developing sewage and waste removal, it was still an age of frequent epidemic disease. The United States met the health challenge by building some 5,000 nonprofit hospitals between 1870 and 1920.* New York gave enormous power to its new state health department to direct the battle against infectious disease. Today, state health departments continue to dominate the healthcare scene in the United States, and hospitals are still the most prominent institutions that the departments regulate.

The history of nursing homes is very different from that of hospitals. Nursing homes evolved out of public asylums as well as from the institutions built and operated by religious and civic groups. It was not until the 1960s and early 1970s that any significant amount of healthcare was introduced into nursing homes. Before then, a home's mission was custodial, based on the assumption that there was little the home could do for older adults except to provide them with safe room and board. Then, in 1965, the creation of Medicaid and Medicare made public funds available for nursing home reimbursement, and the environment changed. The federal government and state departments of health, shaped by their experiences with hospital models, entered to regulate the modern long-term care industry.

In hindsight, it is easy to see that state officials and regulators treated nursing homes as institutional stepchildren in the healthcare family. They viewed long-term care as a kind of hospital variant rather than a separate system. During this era, furthermore, Commissioner Axelrod reshaped the culture of long-term care in New York. He would not allow unequal provisions for the wealthy and the poor; he declared that all residents would be treated equally and an impact would be that their care would be paid predominantly by public funds.

---

* "In 1873 a government survey counted fewer than 200 hospitals. By 1910 over 4000 were counted, and by 1920 more than 6000." (Starr, P. *The social transformation of American medicine: The rise of a sovereign profession and the making of a vast industry.* New York: Basic Books; 1982, 73.)

Based on these principles, the department controlled costs by limiting the percentage of private rooms in nursing homes and the total square footage for which Medicaid would pay. A whole list of requirements followed, including mealtimes, food temperatures, call alarms, fire safety, and many other functions. After paying for all the requirements imposed by the health department, a nursing home had very little discretionary money left.

Standardization and control extended beyond the physical plant. Nursing home clients were vulnerable and unable to advocate for themselves, so over time the Department of Health also set the standards for the training and responsibilities of the long-term care workforce. Because of the state's rigorous inspection process, written documentation of every component of care was required. Eventually, nursing home operations became virtually uniform. Because evidence seemed to show that nursing home residents declined at about the same rate, health policymakers considered the rate of decline in nursing home residents inevitable, predictable, and universal—and assumed this decline was the process of aging itself.

The aging population that the health department seeks to protect is actually diverse, however, and its needs vary widely. The department thus constantly interprets and enforces policy as unforeseen problems arise, filling gaps as it finds them. Despite its determination to set uniform standards, nursing home regulation in New York has become a tangled thicket, a constant swirl of mediation between industry, consumers, trade associations, labor, and legislative interest groups. The same is true in many other states.

Approval Process for the New Home

After years of working with the health department, I came to a very distinct sense of its culture. In order to function in the chaos of competing interests, health department leadership had developed an internal culture that partitioned itself off from the outside world. The shifting sands of legislation, administrative decisions, and judicial rulings were so unstable that the department devised its own scaffolding for decisions, full of internal reasoning that was often not visible to outsiders. Inside the department were well-understood connections between what seemed like unrelated issues. Opaque legal and political matters contained serious policy, financial, and service-delivery consequences. In these circumstances, the department issued decisions that may have seemed arbitrary to providers. Because the logic of its decisions was often hidden, I found it virtually impossible to understand or predict its workings.

Into this mysterious system, we proudly and rather naively carried our new design for what we called our cluster-based nursing home, not realizing at first how we were challenging the assumptions of the powerfully built fortress of the New York State Department of Health. Our simple proposition was that the department's regulatory template for the nursing home no longer addressed the needs of current residents or the tasks of care delivery. We explained patiently that the physical spaces of existing nursing home buildings, although they conformed to department regulations, had imposed routines and living experiences that were actually damaging to the residents.

We pointed out to department regulators that their codes produced bedrooms and bathrooms that were so small that residents were unable to use their residual competencies to get into the bathrooms connected to their bedrooms, which forced them to seek help or to use public facilities. The beds were so close together that even if residents retained the capacity to get into their own wheelchairs and dress themselves, there was insufficient space to do so. In earlier days, this had mattered less because most residents weren't dependent on wheelchairs and could maneuver in a smaller space. As residents had become more frail and their needs had changed, institutional thinking had not adjusted. Everything about aging was changing, and no one was noticing or responding.

We argued that the innovations we were proposing actually extended far beyond the size of bedrooms to the design of the entire platform. If we had truly understood the health department's character at the beginning of the process, we might have been too cowed to ask.

Monthly meetings with the health department went on for a year, then another and another. In Albany, we were shuffled from desk to desk and office to office. What slowly evolved, as we refined our work and sharpened our talk, was an integrated meta-story that we hoped to sell. As already described, our new plan would decentralize the home's functions and do so around the primary relationship between the resident and the nurse's aide. We explained over and over that the resident–aide pairing is the primary factor in care and that the nursing station, a key architectural component of the traditional home, undermines that relationship by pulling the aides away from the residents, leaving them isolated down long corridors. We developed a poster depicting workflow on the new platform, detailing the underlying innovations. Eventually, we presented our ideas to a panel representing all the bureaus in the department, consisting of more than 30 people. Halfway through the presentation, the Head of the Architecture Bureau said, "Mr. Dunkelman, what you are saying is that for the last 10 or 20 years we've been approving the wrong projects." I said, "That's right."

A year later, somewhat miraculously, because of the undeterred efforts of our team, the New Home received a $3 million demonstration grant from the New York State Department of Health. A year after that, the department rewrote its regulations for skilled nursing facilities.

Conclusion

The byzantine nature of health departments continues. If we are going to make more changes to the care system for older adults, it is crucial to be aware of this obstacle to innovation. Our experience in working through the barriers to be able to build the New Home is meant to serve as an example of how a new paradigm can, sometimes with much effort, be achieved.

CHAPTER 6

Confronting the Care System for Older Adults in the United States

Another primary underlying obstacle that inhibited us in designing and implementing our New Home, and a continuing complicating factor in implementing further changes in aging care, is the overall complexity of the current system of care for older adults in the United States. While some families still care for their own older members, additional programs and resources began to supplement family efforts in 20th- and 21st-century America. In addition to nursing homes, national old-age pensions, assisted living, adult day programs, paratransit vehicles, social work, and other services are now a regular part of the landscape.

In fact, we have an extensive configuration of care for older people, analogous to and overlapping our healthcare system. Its interconnecting network includes anything that supports an older man or woman, from Social Security payments to Meals on Wheels delivery to nursing home activities. The system began to take shape in the 1930s during the Great Depression. By now, it consumes more resources than any other area of federal government spending, including the military, as well as a large proportion of state spending.*

Most of us will encounter the system one way or another, perhaps through grandparents or parents and eventually for ourselves. Almost everyone encountering the system finds it baffling. If we understand the system better, maybe we can make later life easier for people, including ourselves, when it is our turn. The more we know about our single largest tax-supported expense, furthermore, the better our chances of avoiding costly policy blunders.

---

*Here is a breakdown of government spending in 2019: Social Security, $1 trillion; Medicare, $644 billion; Medicaid, $409 billion, for a total $2.052 trillion. Total federal healthcare spending was $4.4 trillion; defense spending was $676 billion. (Statistics from "The Federal Budget in 2019: An Infographic," Congressional Budget Office, April 15, 2020, https://www.cbo.gov/publication/56324.)

It's easier to find separate parts of the system of care for older adults than to see the totality of it. There is no well-marked front door or usable directory. In fact, it's easy to think there is no connected system at all. It's essentially invisible from the outside because inside it is a vast maze. No direct routes can be seen from one point to the next, and the organization is as opaque to the uninitiated as the tax code. A relatively small matter can serve as an illustrative example: If a client needs durable medical equipment, he or she is covered by Medicare Part B while at home. If the client is then hospitalized under Medicare Part A or goes to a long-term care facility, the coverage for a new wheelchair stops.

Sources of care for older adults are often not connected to one another. Even though the different programs were initiated and developed independently, there was sufficient flexibility at first so that handoffs from one level of care to the next could occur naturally as people's needs changed. However, as hospitals, nursing homes, and assisted living centers have tightened the services they offer, what used to be an integrated system for long-term care has broken down. Because these facilities are so specialized, there is no longer sufficient overlap between levels of care, and no time is spent on planning and transitioning older clients smoothly from one institution to another. The easy byways connecting the facilities for aging care have been cut, resulting in separate islands that have no bridges to one another.

The character of aging policy in the United States is a product of our history, our national character, and even our geography. The various programs and resources that have been developed for aging care can appear very alien to each other because there was never a comprehensive plan for a unified policy. Today's system was created by separate efforts to cope with aging care, as well as by features of our national life that are unrelated to aging, including our attitudes toward government, politics, science, and organizational behavior. No one person or group decided to build the system we have. It began with traditional governmental responses to social issues at particular moments in history and then developed under the influence of cultural elements and unanticipated consequences.

What follows is a thumbnail account of how current confusing policies for aging came to be in the United States. It is really two intertwined stories. One is about how and why programs developed, and the other describes how features of our national landscape influenced the specifics of the buildings we have chosen to construct.

History of Aging Care Policy in the United States

Two circumstances changed life for older adults in the United States during the second half of the 19th century. One was the westward expansion of the population. Younger generations began moving toward the frontier in the early 1800s, leaving their parents behind and on their own. Second, industrialization and urbanization created a fundamental change for older men and women. Cities were much less hospitable to the traditional ways of caring for the older members of a family than rural life had been. Families who moved into cities from farms were less able to keep multiple generations in one dwelling or to benefit from having an aging parent to help with tasks. On the farm, an older worker's jobs simply shrank as his or her powers declined, but in the world of factories, when the worker's powers declined, his or her productivity disappeared.

At first, the government provided services to older adults only when they were also poor. During much of the 19th century, people with no way to get by went into the poorhouse, where they were housed with alcoholics, individuals with disabilities, orphans, petty criminals, and people with mental illness. Late in the century, religious and fraternal groups, early labor unions, and immigrant community associations built "old folks' homes" for their older members, who either paid their way in as subscribers or were provided for by fellow immigrants. Unlike modern facilities for older people, the 19th-century old folks' home was not regulated.

At the start of the 20th century, it became increasingly apparent that older adults might need separate consideration as a class of their own. New York City turned its largest poorhouse, filled primarily with sick older men and women, into an infirmary for the aged. In the late 1920s, states began to provide welfare for indigent older people.

The severity of the Great Depression caused a fundamental rethinking of social welfare as a national responsibility. Because the economic collapse was so pervasive, it stripped poverty of the moral stigma of individual failure. The economic calamity inspired a federal commitment to welfare for individual citizens and a change in attitude toward poverty, particularly in older age. More than half the states had old-age relief programs in place by the mid-1930s. In 1935, passage of the Social Security Act created the first national program of assistance for older Americans. It included Old Age Assistance, a program that matched federal money with the welfare payments 28 states were already making to the older poor, and it took effect immediately. This initiated the principle, still in existence, that the next generation pays for the previous one.

In 1950, the federal government started making direct reimbursements to medical vendors who treated welfare recipients. In 1960, Medical Assistance for the Aged was introduced, creating a federal program for people over 65 who did not qualify for welfare but were nonetheless facing larger medical expenses than they could afford. At the same time, Congress created low-income housing programs for older adults and grants for building nursing homes.

By 1960, in the 25 years since the passage of the Social Security Act, the federal government had also become directly involved with the healthcare of low- and moderate-income older adults and with the housing of low-income older adults. In 1965, two amendments to the Social Security Act created Medicare and Medicaid. A third piece of legislation, the Older Americans Act, completed the framework of our present system of care for advancing age. Although elements of these programs had been under discussion since the early 1900s, when our (still) elusive idea of universal health insurance was first proposed, there had been little to indicate that such a revolutionary change in healthcare financing could ever be accomplished. This leap in 1965 into a new order of social welfare is still breathtaking in its suddenness and scope. In a few summer weeks, Congress enacted universal single-payer health insurance for everyone 65 and older (Medicare), a comprehensive medical welfare program for poor people of all ages (Medicaid), and a package of programs to assist older adults in other ways (the Older Americans Act). Nothing remotely comparable in government-sponsored social policy has happened in the more than half-century since. The Affordable Care Act of 2010, while significant, simply extends the programs established in 1965 to more recipients.

The original Social Security Act of 1935 is the only existing old age–related program of equivalent magnitude, and it was created in response to the national disaster of the Great Depression. Medicare,

Medicaid, and the Older Americans Act resulted from a burst of high hopes that the programs would shore up a weakness in our social fabric and rescue older men and women from destitution, homelessness, hunger, and lack of medical care. It was a noble undertaking meant to create social programs that make advanced age at least safe and comfortable for almost everyone. Our current aging programs did not evolve slowly and incrementally with widespread understanding and recognition by the underlying populace, but out of suddenly passed, specifically focused laws.

The new legislation of the mid-1960s still determines the way we approach programming for older adults. Our legislatures have subsequently inserted particular programs to deal with additional needs of older people as they emerge, beginning with funds to deal with poverty in late life, then support for medical and custodial expenses, followed by subsidies for housing, transportation, and meals. We have separate programs to deal with each of these needs rather than a system that approaches the needs of our oldest citizens holistically.

Once created, each program developed on its own, driven by a combination of the realities of advancing age, the programs' own internal dynamics, and some external circumstances such as medical breakthroughs. We have not revisited the original designs of Medicare, Medicaid, and the Older Americans Act, even though the late phase of life today is not what it was 50 years ago. We talk about reform, but we have not acted. We use the existing system, oil it, patch it up, and accept it as a fundamental part of life in the United States. Until recently, the proportion of the population that was elderly was small enough for issues of aging to have little role in our national discourse.

Americanism of Aging Care Policy in the United States

Our aging support programs have been shaped at least as much by some specific features of the unique history and character of the United States as by the needs of older adults. Our current aging care–delivery system reflects how older age has wended its way through 250 years of U.S. history, and, over the last 75 years, through the constitutional, legislative, and free-enterprise framework of the United States. How America experiences old age is at least in part a product of this unique history. Sometimes the landscape of modern aging appears to be almost perversely irrational. In order to move forward, it is critical to understand how the historical foundations of our national system for aging care continue to shape it.

The first and most fundamental influence on our aging enterprise is that the nation is a federation of states. As a result, we have ended up with 50 aging policies, not one, even though some of them are federal. Second, our government divides and balances power among the legislative, executive, and judicial branches. Third, our free-enterprise economy plays a role in shaping aging policy. Much more than anything inherent in aging itself, these fundamental realities have determined how our policies toward aging work. Trying to understand programs for aging from the perspective of the needs of older adults won't make sense without first understanding why the complications, restrictions, and the lack of coordination between services exist. By looking at how the United States makes policy, programs for aging may be easier to understand, even if what they produce is unwieldy from the consumer's point of view.

Federalism

The early European immigrants to the New World were escaping the oppression of kings and church. Our Constitution and Bill of Rights were framed to protect 13 separate sovereign states from federal authority. In domestic matters, the federal government is often a creature of the states. It is sometimes helpful to think of the United States as 50 different countries that are oddly alike but nonetheless different and sovereign. There is always some resistance to any federal role in state business. This tension is as old as the nation. With aging, the sovereignty of the states is not a minor technicality. When Social Security was created in 1935, one of its provisions was that the federal government would pay half the cost of states' welfare programs for the aged poor (this eventually evolved to become Medicaid, as described below), requiring the states to bear part of the burden if they wanted federal money.[†] It would only be available, furthermore, to states that started

---

[†] There was early state–federal sharing of responsibility with Social Security. When Social Security became a totally federal responsibility, Medicaid continued the pattern of shared federal–state responsibility.

old-age welfare eligibility by age 65, rather than later. Medicare, on the other hand, follows an alternative path. It is a purely federal program through which every U.S. citizen over 65 who has paid into the system is entitled to healthcare coverage without regard to income.

Medicaid, the third major program, works out its federal and state relationship in a manner entirely unlike either Social Security or Medicare. Because it was designed as a state–federal program from the beginning, each state has a say in how its program works. Medicaid only covers people with incomes or assets below specified levels. When the states' representatives in Congress wrote the Medicaid statute, they allowed each state to decide whether or not it wanted to involve itself and made federal support for the state programs proportional to the wealth of the state, with the federal share being 50% of the costs for the richest states, and up to 85% for poorer states. This was a compromise between rich states that wanted the matching program and poor states that didn't want to pay for the rich states' programs. This political reality shaped Medicaid. The legislation had more to do with the architecture of our division into states than with needs intrinsic to aging.

The state–federal arrangement makes every paragraph in each state's Medicaid system a complicated negotiation. State programs reflect the individual state's political climate and culture. Some states even transfer responsibility to the county level so that negotiations on what services the program covers may be three levels deep, from federal, to state, to county. Changing administrations at both the state and federal level have changing views on what to encourage or discourage.

In New York, as in many states, Medicaid consumes almost 50% of the state budget and, in addition to that, about one-third of the budgets of New York's counties.[30] Not all of this goes to older adults—Medicaid covers the poor of all ages—but an increasingly large and fast-growing proportion does. Because states have different policies and because the state–federal Medicaid share formula is different from state to state, not every state bears such heavy Medicaid expenses, but many do.

The individual agreements between states and the federal government under the Medicaid program have become bewilderingly diverse and complex. In practice, the long-term care system of the nation follows 50 different sets of rules. Some states are more generous than others toward older people in need. Some regulate programs more intensively. Some have relatively younger or older populations. Across all of these variations, federal Medicaid program managers must negotiate contracts that are reasonably equitable to different states while also allowing them some flexibility. So federalism, our fundamental national constitutional arrangement, is a key determinant of the experience of older age in this country. To understand aging in the United States, it is crucial to understand our federalized system.

Branches of Government

The way programs for older adults are actually administered is another crucial factor in how our care system works. The programs are written and enacted by elected officials, but their day-to-day administration is the province of managers within government agencies. Congress, for example, may pass a law to subsidize rent-controlled housing for people 62 and older, but administrators in the Department of Housing and Urban Development actually commission the buildings. Their decisions can sometimes be contradictory to the needs of the people they serve. For example, as individuals who live in subsidized apartment buildings grow older, they may need structural accommodations for their wheelchairs or easier access to additional medical services. The agency might see those modifications as threats to its budget or its regulatory prerogatives. This organizational reality, which may have nothing to do with aging, plays a large part in determining if, when, where, and how aging services will be delivered in a given state.

The federal legislation of 1965 started several programs from scratch, directing that each address specific needs for certain older men and women in particular settings. Both the program managers in federal and state offices and the older people they serve have representatives monitoring the programs. Governmental administrators who want to keep their programs going must ensure that only the target population is included in a given program and that those outside of that population are excluded, even if some would benefit from it. At points where their programs come into contact, such as when a transportation service to a senior center interfaces with a meals program at the same center, their separate fortress walls could spring a leak. The transportation administrator may be concerned that funds dedicated to transportation will be used inappropriately by beneficiaries of other services who are not themselves eligible for the transportation program. As another example, a manager of a housing program for independent seniors may ignore unauthorized homecare services being brought into the building so that he or she does not lose clients.

Up and down the funding chain, agency administrators, providers, older adults, and others negotiate the details and boundaries of programs. Judicial interaction with the care system adds another layer of complication to the management of the program, one that is intensified by unpredictability. Court rulings, like software patches, can have unintended consequences. When confronted with an older person whose dire circumstances could be relieved if an apparently arbitrary regulation were revised, a judge might kindly extend the program to the person appearing before him or her, thus unwittingly opening the entire program to a new class of beneficiaries. Such a judgment can play havoc with the program's budget and cause it to evolve in an unanticipated direction. If a case changes the eligibility requirements for an individual in assisted living, it may make the new requirements available to everyone. This shift might attract residents away from another program that in turn collapses because its expected target population is smaller than anticipated and it loses funding. Allowing coverage for a wheelchair for one plaintiff could change federal policy to mean that wheelchairs have to be supplied to thousands of clients, which will have a major effect on the durable medical equipment industry. As programs evolve, the case law around them becomes extraordinarily complex and arcane. Under pressure from aggrieved parties seeking judicial relief, the care system for older adults has been repeatedly patched and rewritten in ways that are obscure even to professionals in aging care, particularly when the change is in a program several silos away.

In summary, the aging policies created by the individual states and the federal government are interpreted by the legislative branches and then executed by bureaucrats who translate legislative policy into practice. The policies and their implementation are further subject to change by the judicial branch. This is not the simplest or quickest way to design aging care programs, but it is the way we do it in the United States.

Private Sector

Describing the whirling world of aging care policymaking and program management still doesn't reveal how the care reaches older adults. In almost all instances, government programs pay for aging care services rather than providing them directly. That responsibility is handed over to private enterprise. Government programs supply the money that pays for a service, defines its scope, sets its standards, and sometimes licenses vendors to deliver specified services to older people, such as homecare or daycare. Medicare pays medical bills for anyone older than 65 who has paid in, but doctors in private practice provide the actual care. The federal government provides low-interest loans and other subsidies for low-income housing for older adults, and a government department commissions the construction, but private developers build it.

The private vendors and businesses that actually provide the services have a fundamental interest in making the enterprise work. The actual delivery of aging care is made up of companies, both for-profit and nonprofit, that want to stay in operation. They need office space, employees, equipment, bookkeeping, and a bank account. They look for a steady stream of clients to serve and a steady stream of funds. Yet, both the client stream and the funding streams may ebb and flow. The provider plans to work with a specific category of clients, funding streams, and regulatory structures, but the target client may move to a different program or the government may reduce funding. Perhaps a new regulation or a new court decision imposes new requirements that force a provider to seek out different clients, invest in building renovations, or retrain different staff. What may look like a growing and stable market from the outside because the number of older adults is swelling is actually a rollercoaster ride for the provider.

Aging care providers are focused on survival as much as service, as are their counterparts in the government bureaus that administer aging programs. From outside, it may appear that the bureaucracy and the providers are unresponsive, but they are actually hyper-vigilant about policy interpretations and potential issues on the periphery that could affect them. The government regulators and the service providers conduct a continuous negotiation, which intertwines with the complications in the care system for older people arising from federalism in the United States, from the behavior of the bureaucracies that implement the rules, and from the intervention of courts. There is minimal incentive or residual energy to find the least expensive and least invasive option for the older person or to fill the cracks and smooth the rough edges of programs overwhelmed by the changes in the aging population. Common sense and flexibility cannot play the roles we wish they could because they get lost in the system.

Conclusion

Since 1965, the basic tenets of the programs for aging have not changed significantly, but aging itself has changed a great deal. The changes, including the lengthening of life and the engagement of government in so many aspects of aging—not to mention the impact of chronic conditions that will be discussed at length later on—have all compounded into the current chaotic state of the delivery of aging care. No one part of the system looks at the overall status of the older person. The result on the ground for consumers is that they experience a blizzard of changing programs that are difficult to combine into an integrated care plan offering any sense of security. Getting a van to take a parent to congregate meals, scheduling homecare services, and filling medications may require three entirely separate providers with different administrative rules. Attempting to orchestrate a frail person's day through this labyrinth wears out the most assiduous caring son or daughter and often leaves the frail older adult confused and even at risk.

The tensions on a family can compound. The Medicaid nursing home bed everyone expected may not be accessible, for even if a parent is very frail, he or she may not sufficiently or appropriately meet the regulations for admission. If the person does find a bed, the nursing home itself may have become ever more unsatisfying from lack of funding. The voices rising in complaint become ever more shrill, clamoring for all-encompassing change. Blame is placed on deadlocked legislatures, incompetent bureaucracies, unresponsive courts, inefficient and greedy providers, thankless children abandoning their parents, or even on older people themselves, who now live too long and are devouring the future. Sadly, this anger and confusion created by our disjointed system of caring for older adults just pushes us further from the new realities of aging and the abundant opportunities for making this a time of life as meaningful as every other.

CHAPTER 7

Aging Care Meets
the Changing World

Three great changes came to the world of aging in the United States in the 20th century, as we have seen: the conquering of many infectious diseases along with advances in public health; the creation of Social Security, Medicare, Medicaid, and the Older Americans Act; and the growth of long-term care for older adults into a large industry, provided primarily by nursing homes. These changes have resulted in many older men and women who continue to live after becoming very frail, in massive governmental involvement in aging, and in the rise of an industrial complex to provide care for the rapidly growing aging population. It is clear that we need to find better ways to address this brand-new universe than the ones we have now. The New Home was an attempt to find a solution, even though our progress was slowed down by the maze of regulations and by the byzantine complexity of the existing care system for older people in the United States.

Beyond the New Home

We designed the New Home to preserve the dignity of our residents and make life agreeable for them. We had encouragement from a progressive board of directors and financial support from our community. Our ambition was more than local. If we got it right, we thought, we could demonstrate a way out of the traditional physical designs and care routines that were causing so many older adults so much distress. Our hopes even went beyond disseminating our New Home model. When the New Home was up and running, we saw that we had successfully created spaces and systems that freed our residents from some of the unfortunate consequences of old-style institutional care. We had transformed the unhappy lives of many nursing home residents, who had no privacy and spent long hours in their wheelchairs waiting for bathrooms, meals, and activities. Until the New Home, that Industrial Age line model was the only known answer to the problem of how to keep a profoundly frail older person alive and safe. With the New Home, we had made a radical change from old-style care, moving from a system that had to be rigid to function into an organization that made flexibility its basic operating principle. After its success, it was tempting to continue to see if we could reform other kinds of old-age care. Were there possibilities to meet older people's needs that were even less institutional than a nursing home, even one as nice as ours? We wanted to go further on the road to providing modernized care for older adults. We started asking ourselves to consider whether all nursing home residents belonged in such facilities in the first place. We wondered what other kinds of care we could develop for the much larger population of frail older Americans who were not in nursing homes.

After building and operating the New Home, making corrections and adjustments, and delivering 10 years of single-minded effort, we realized the cluster form of management and the approaches to care we had developed around it would not be scalable to the expanding size of the population arriving onto the scene. It also became apparent that societal conditions and assumptions about aging had changed so significantly that the New Home, successful as it was, was already little more than an interesting model with limited application. Was it a good solution to a truly awful set of problems at the time we built it? Yes. Was it worth the effort, even if it wasn't a final answer? Absolutely. But the New Home couldn't deliver on its promise because its capacity was too limited and its individual price too high in relation to the growing demand that was slowly becoming visible. Aging had simply overflowed the dikes and flooded the existing care system for older adults.

The model created in the New Home worked. Almost 30 years later, it still works as a facility to house and care for frail older residents in comfort and dignity—but I wouldn't build another one myself. I no longer believe that even an excellently run, appropriately designed long-term care institution is the right place for a large proportion of frail older people.

The range of differences among older adults increases with age. This goes against a common misperception that all older people are alike. The differences among them have great significance for the design of buildings for them. It is to be hoped that the dramatically increasing number of frail older men and women will enable us to design and populate many specialized settings, with associated programs, protocols, and staff training.

That is at the center of what this book is about. In the future, facilities like the New Home, perhaps on a smaller scale, might be a nice niche offering in an upscale retirement community. Our innovations, however, are not the answer to the broader question of how to care for large numbers of frail older adults who are arriving on the scene. In the New Home, we answered more narrowly framed concerns about how to redesign care routines in a nursing home to improve each resident's quality of life. We had to figure out how to balance design, cost, and quality care while staying in business. We did not address the bigger question posed by the dramatic changes in society I have described previously: How can we meet the care needs of the many millions of frail people who are approaching their 90s?

During the years we were developing and building the New Home and the years we spent refining our organization and care routines, additional circumstances beyond our purview at the time were changing rapidly, leaving our model stranded. The greatest shift was in the profile of our residents, caused by modifications in public policy. The gathering forces I have described in earlier chapters—the demographics of aging, the challenge of providing care for extended years, the cost of that care to the state—began to exert downward pressure on nursing homes, forcing the less frail residents to make way for older and more frail ones. I will describe that pressure and its results in a moment, but it is important to keep in mind that as a consequence, slightly healthier older people who previously might have entered the New Home as a safe place to spend the last years of their lives now needed an alternative: either a way to stay at home or the option of a different kind of residence that accommodated their needs. They wouldn't need to be housed in a skilled nursing facility.

We explored many options. We introduced a version of community living into the New Home, with its private, semiprivate, and public spaces, and became increasingly mindful of the community outside our walls. Maybe we could blend some of our residents, the ones who did not need continual nursing care, back into a community setting. Or perhaps the New Home, as we had conceived it for residents with a particular range of abilities, was itself unnecessary if we could divide its residents into those living in residential neighborhoods and those who were very frail and required more attention. It was an interesting puzzle, with each question evoking answers that provoked further questions.

We weren't the only ones thinking about this, of course. By the time we got the New Home up and running, the world of care for aging adults had for some years been energetically creating and commercializing a variety of informal care possibilities. Nursing homes were already being supplemented by a variety of other living arrangements that were coming onto the scene. Many of these new options, such as assisted living facilities and continuing care retirement communities, were understood to be way stations between private residences and nursing homes. As I will describe later, we expanded into these areas ourselves. We created an organization to deliver in-home care. We built subsidized housing for low-income seniors. We created a first-of-its-kind combination apartment house and wraparound frailty care program for mostly poor older adults, all of whom would have been in nursing homes if they had not been in our program. If a concept offered a way to provide care or support for older people, especially those approaching frailty or who were already frail, we tried it. In addition to the New Home, we assembled on and off our campus working models of all the major responses to aging care available at the beginning of the 21st century, all in a search for broader solutions commensurate with the looming population that would need help in its old age.

The Evolution of Medicaid and Its Impact on Nursing Homes

One of our motivations for exploring alternative solutions for aging care was, as I have indicated, the inability of nursing homes to provide an adequate answer to the changing problems of older-age care. This issue can be traced back to the 1965 creation of Medicaid, which provides healthcare insurance for the poor and, importantly, covers long-term care costs for people who can't afford it. Based on the predominant Industrial Age thinking at the time of its creation, Medicaid shaped the long-term care industry we know today. At first, the program stimulated an intensive expansion of long-term care institutions by providing a reliable source of funding. As already described, the funding came with increasingly intense regulation by federal and state governments, including crucial new rules about who could receive assistance. The rules were complicated and they varied from state to state, but because the federal government was now paying at least 50% of the cost states could improve services for their poorer aging citizens at half price or less. In some states, Medicaid also affected the delivery of long-term care by paying more for services delivered in nursing homes than for those delivered to private homes, making nursing home care a more financially attractive alternative to older adults and their families. In those states nursing homes boomed.

In its early years, Medicaid paid for long-term care at one set daily rate. The care consisted largely of making comfortable those people who couldn't take care of themselves in their last years, but some residents and some conditions were more expensive to address than others. Furthermore, some people could and would privately pay a higher amount for care than the Medicaid flat rate. That led nursing homes to give precedence to such privately paying clients over Medicaid recipients, and to prefer healthier older residents for whom care was less expensive. The government, too, preferred having clients who paid on their own, enabling Medicaid to reimburse the nursing home for a smaller number of clients and forcing the institution to charge the private payer more in order to balance its own budget.

Of course, private payers quickly figured out the cost shifting that was being implemented at their expense. In order to take proper advantage of the intricacies of the rules, a corner of the legal profession developed the specialty of elder law, finding ways to enable the middle class to transfer a family member's money to his or her descendants, thus making the older family member eligible for Medicaid. In other words, middle-class older adults found ways to become artificially poor so they could access government funds. What was designed as a program for the very poor became, effectively, an entitlement for the middle class. This was not consistent with the original legislative intent of the Medicaid program.

The problem created by facilities favoring healthier applicants over more frail ones was finally addressed in the early 1990s, when we were building the New Home. The New York State Department of Health planners began to appreciate the scale and needs of the growing population of the very frail. New digital data collection and analysis allowed health departments to measure variables in care and predict outcomes. The old flat-rate reimbursement, which encouraged homes to accept healthier applicants and refuse admission to the more frail, was finally recognized as bad public policy.

Refining the Nursing Home Population

In an attempt to find a better system, policymakers produced studies showing that a few basic variables, such as how well a frail person walked or used the toilet, could accurately predict how much overall care he or she required. Levels of need were called Resource Utilization Groups, or RUGs. They defined how many resources a particular resident required. The Department of Health developed a standard form for evaluating each resident in a nursing home, averaged the scores, and derived a "facility score" to determine how much the state would pay that facility for the daily care of each of its Medicaid recipients.

The RUG system created a financial incentive to admit frailer older adults rather than healthier ones. At first, there was a kind of gold rush to admit the frailest clients, but nursing homes soon recognized that the costs associated with the frailest residents exceeded even the most generous payments on the Medicaid scale. For maximum financial efficiency, nursing homes began to specialize by grouping residents by specific need levels.

Nursing homes soon developed their own computer programs to evaluate candidates and, beyond that, to identify every person's limitations in order to nudge residents into higher scoring categories that would bring in higher reimbursements from Medicaid. A facility had a financial incentive for its residents to become frailer so that their reimbursement value would rise, while assuring that the residents did not deteriorate so quickly that the state would suspect a failure of care. The state started to monitor each resident's status online to look for statistical discrepancies, such as residents losing function at a suspiciously high rate, which would then enable the state to fine the home and recoup reimbursement.

Although it took a few years to train the nursing home staff to collect multiple variables on each resident and to accumulate them into a facility score, homes did so for their own financial best interests. The nursing home could no longer afford to care for residents who were less frail and would thus pull down its overall reimbursement rate. As the frailty of the population increased, the organization had to hire specialized staff and purchase more sophisticated equipment, creating higher costs and making it even more critical that the residents be classified as more frail under the RUG Medicaid reimbursement system.

For the state, there are a number of benefits to the RUG system, which is still in effect. First, the system functions as a triaging mechanism encouraging care for frailty. This is a reasonable policy goal, and it has the additional benefit of appearing to be based on a system through which results can be measured and monitored. The financial incentives embedded in a RUG system also lead to shorter nursing home stays. As homes admit frailer clients with shorter life expectancies, the length of stay of residents has plummeted. At one time, the length of stay in a nursing home was about 8.5 years; today it is likely to be less than 6 months.

Furthermore, by using RUGs, the Department of Health can constantly jiggle reimbursement categories, incentivizing and disincentivizing care for whole categories of people. One of the consequences of this system, however, is that nursing homes have become an aging care option that is far from universally applicable. Nursing homes have assumed a character closer to that of hospital care, taking on the sights, sounds, and smells of a hospital. They have also become less attractive as places for middle-class families with an aging parent who needs some assistance but is not extremely frail. Because the nursing home is dramatically more expensive for private payers, other residential and community options have now become more appealing to people with money. This, in turn, is hard on middle-class families.

The Rise of Assisted Living

As the population of nursing homes has shifted from younger, more capable clients to older, frailer residents who need more services, the demand for alternatives has grown. With the RUG system in place, the next logical choice for frail older adults who do not yet qualify for nursing homes is assisted living.

Beginning in the late 1980s, a series of simplistic architectural models mesmerized the aging care industry and took shape in variations on an assisted living model. A range of solutions was announced, one after another, with great fanfare. Inevitably their unresponsiveness to the underlying nature and needs of frailty was revealed. Their effectiveness was also blunted by government regulations that sought to align the new facilities with their intended clients' profiles. These circumstances raised the costs of the enterprises while deflating the hope that they could be an all-purpose substitute for nursing home care.

In the early 1990s, for example, long-term care for older people was viewed as a natural offshoot of the hospitality industry. It took a decade to realize that traditional hospitality programs do not appropriately serve frail clients. Older adults need specialized aging services. After the departure of the hospitality industry by about 2000, big investors in the nursing home business took their turn to find a kind of assisted living that could serve as an alternative to nursing homes. They suggested that some levels of frailty could be addressed less expensively and with more dignity in apartment settings. The working premise, not unreasonably, was that the nursing home itself had contributed to the limitations of its frail residents and that, once released from overly institutionalized and regulated environments, many disabilities would evaporate or be dramatically mitigated. The frail older man or woman would return to an earlier, more independent level of functioning. In the New Home, I also fell victim, to some extent, to this overly optimistic, overly generalized thinking when we saw residents who did indeed function better in our new setting. In truth, it is difficult to predict just how much of a frail older person's difficulties are reversible.

Early assisted living buildings often reduced costs by employing designs and construction that were actually antagonistic to the needs of frail adults. The least expensive design for a residential building is a rectangular shape, with long narrow corridors lined with apartments. Such assisted living facilities often presented a breathtaking entrance, an inviting public living room, and an elegant—although often undersized—dining room. This early design oversized personal space in the apartments, making it difficult for the frail resident to manage his or her most immediate tasks, and offered no relaxed semipublic space. It also created long distances to travel to the dining room and the public spaces.

A key objective in the care of frail older adults is to observe the residents in order to head off downward physical and emotional spirals. When occupants are isolated in their apartments because the building is difficult to navigate, they are at increased risk. Long corridors and outsized rooms also increase the staff time needed to transport residents to meals and public spaces, which in turn increases costs. The additional expense may challenge the organization's financial sustainability. There are a few possible organizational responses: pass the cost along to residents in higher rents, thereby limiting the potential resident pool to wealthy people, or hold the line on cost by staffing at an inadequate level. Insisting on standardized ratios of aides to clients does not always fulfill the changing needs of frail adults. Workable staffing ratios depend on a dynamic between the physical environment and the level of the resident's functioning.

Experience eventually demonstrated the importance of designing assisted living facilities around the actual profiles of frail residents. The idea that the nursing home was causing the frailty all by itself turned out to be naïve. Many of the early assisted living buildings didn't address the actual characteristics of their residents. So, some nursing home residents could be successfully transferred to assisted living, but many others, as I'll explain later, found the new situations unworkable. For nursing home residents without means, furthermore, assisted living was not an alternative, even if it would have been appropriate, because Medicaid and other government assistance programs would not pay for it. So, nursing homes, now more medicalized, remained full of very frail older adults, and the new assisted living facilities filled up with slightly less frail older people from the community who had financial means. Neither option served slightly less frail individuals who were also poor.

Design, programming, and care in some more recent assisted living facilities have evolved to meet actual needs better. As the reality of resident needs has manifested itself, family and consumer concerns have grown and governmental investigation has led to higher regulation. After a decade of trial and error, more mature models of assisted living facilities have emerged. Rather than being seen as a less expensive alternative to long-term care that might even eliminate the need for nursing homes, assisted living now offers much more limited benefits to a smaller constituency than originally imagined. Many facilities have developed their own specializations to serve different degrees of frailty and different types of physical and cognitive loss. Appropriately designed and programmed assisted living is a viable option for some frail older adults for some period of their lives, but, again, it is not a universal solution.

On our campus, for example, after we came to realize that the New Home was not the answer to every problem, we created several different kinds of assisted living. We built apartments that use nursing home bathroom design specifications, anticipating that the buildings' residents would eventually be in wheelchairs and should not be forced to leave because of the change. We also offered the option of bringing homecare into the apartments so that very frail people could continue to live in them even after they needed assistance. We built a more intensive assisted living facility, known in New York State as an *adult home*, for a level of care situated somewhere between a nursing home room and an assisted living apartment. Each of these alternatives worked well in itself, but none looked like the wave of the future in care for the aging.

Assisted living provides an opportunity to transfer some less frail older adults to less expensive settings, leaving frailer individuals in nursing homes. As the length of stay shortened in assisted living facilities and costs rose, assisted living turned out to be an alternative available only to the middle class, perhaps only to the upper middle class. That leaves two-thirds of the older population still waiting at the gates.

Small-Scale Nursing Homes

In addition to assisted living, there has been some enthusiasm for a simplified design for aging care that has been applied to small-scale nursing homes, those with 24–48 beds. They are built to resemble elegant homes and to be integrated as much as possible into the surrounding neighborhoods. With large, gracious living rooms and carpeted bedroom suites, every design and program element is calibrated to declare independence and luxury, supported by nursing care. They eschew the institutional atmosphere of larger facilities.

Appealing as this may sound, the packaging again imposes characteristics that clash with the challenge of frailty.

As with much assisted living, the first problem of small-scale homes is the physical design. The quest to create more independence can push private bedroom spaces away from the vaunted great rooms, ironically re-creating, if on a smaller scale, the problematic corridors of the old-style nursing homes. The distant great room, which in this design usually combines kitchen, dining, laundry, and social spaces, as well as tables for activities and communication, becomes a magnet for staff. It would take superhuman resistance for aides not to feel enticed away from the residents' rooms, where frail residents spend their time, in order to join colleagues who are busy at more interesting social chores. Finally, with such a small number of residents, there is insufficient activity in the community space to create the variety necessary to sustain a client's social needs, which are an important part of emotional health. The scale is also too small for separate support departments, so the duties of nurse's aide, dietary aide, housekeeper, and launderer are usually combined into a universal worker. This can set up a competitive dynamic between the universal worker's people-oriented tasks (helping residents in the bathroom, answering call bells, assisting residents with dressing) and his or her mechanical tasks (laundry, cleaning, kitchen chores). The mechanical tasks take place in socially engaging spaces around the great room, in the company of fellow employees. Workers often come to prefer them to the more private, boring, perhaps unpleasant people care tasks, distant from the fun and stimulation.

Another difficulty built into the design of small-scale nursing homes arises from its apparent principal virtue: the small number of older adults in the facility. A limited client base may not generate sufficient revenue to hire and retain caregivers with the sophisticated expertise and judgment required for the care of today's frail older people. There is insufficient client volume, for example, for a doctor to visit frequently enough to develop strong relationships with the care team. The small scale may not attract supervisors with the necessary expertise because highly qualified nurse supervisors prefer higher paying jobs in larger settings. There may be inadequate observation of residents' physical status. The challenge to maintain adequate supervision becomes greatest in the evening, when there is minimal staffing and residents are tired, less strong, less alert, and more at risk for accidents.

Small-scale settings also inherently do not favor the best individualized care for frail older adults. There are insufficient numbers of residents in each facility to develop deep specialization in care. If the small setting selects a niche in which to specialize, a person whose needs change from the specialty runs the risk of being stranded in an environment no longer fitted to his or her needs. The small-scale home can easily evolve into a beautifully appointed setting, doing a bit of this and that, none of it well.

PACE Program

Assisted living alternatives turn out to be, for the most part, only available to people with comfortable financial means. Our aging care organization, however, wanted to offer services for all the oldest members of our community who needed us. Our mission impelled us to look for ways to provide alternatives to frail persons with little or no means. We found PACE (Program for All-inclusive Care for the Elderly).

The Basic Premise of PACE-Capitated Frailty

In the early 1970s, the Chinese community in San Francisco created an adult day program for older adults living in their area. Over the next decade, it added nurse's aides, transportation, and a physician, and became On Lok Senior Health Services. It extended these coordinated services into the homes of its clients when necessary. The program's managers came to realize that without these services virtually all their clients might have to enter nursing homes. So, they proposed to the state of California that if the state would pay them 70% of the nursing home reimbursement rate for each of their clients, they would take on the responsibility for the client's care and not expect any further support from the state. If a client had to be moved into a nursing home, the program would pay the nursing home's full rate and would continue to accept 70% of that rate from the government.

After coming to this agreement with the state, On Lok went to the federal government, which agreed to a 70% monthly prepayment for Medicare on the same basis. This was an early example of what is called *capitation* in healthcare, the payment of a monthly premium per head to an agency that would then be responsible for whatever health expenses its enrollees required. The federal government agreed to partner with California's Medicaid program, called Medi-Cal, and to extend Medicare benefits on a capitated basis to On Lok participants. So On Lok had a guaranteed revenue stream with which to keep its old, often frail clientele cared for. The program managers also had a powerful incentive to keep their clients healthy because they were at risk for the entire cost of each client's healthcare. The program itself, as devised between On Lok and its government payers, was quite strict. Clients continued to live at home but were required to make frequent visits to a day center, where an interdisciplinary team planned services and care as needed for each member.

The program demonstrated that frail older adults could stay safely in their communities for dramatically less cost than in a nursing home, and with less disruption to their lives. It also demonstrated that, at least for the population in San Francisco's Chinese community, an organization could reduce risks by following very thoughtful care routines and intervening quickly to prevent cascading problems. Its arrangement extended Medicaid payments beyond the walls of the nursing home, a feature critical to the future of care for the aging. Because of its success, PACE was given Demonstration Status by the federal government, enabling other states to develop it.

Our Venture into the PACE Program

When New York State approved the model, we decided to introduce it to the Buffalo area. We went to PACE conferences and studied the few existing programs. It was a dramatically innovative concept that seemed very foreign to many older adults and their families. It had to compete with familiar and well-established nursing homes and homecare agencies that were adept at selecting and capturing appropriate candidates. It was hard for people to grasp the fact that PACE would be more cost-effective and offer more security because it took care of people even as their needs evolved.

It was clear that a multiyear process would be required to operationalize a PACE program and break even. We would have to begin building enrollment slowly with the more complex and expensive clients that the homecare agencies and nursing homes did not want. The program would have to hire a full retinue of staff even though the program might start with only one participant. It could take several years to get enough participants to cover costs. We calculated that our PACE was likely to accumulate $3–$5 million in losses in its first few years, with little prospect of recouping them in the following years.

We simply did not have the resources to absorb such a large loss—but our aging community would clearly benefit from a PACE program. If we were going to have one, we would have to cut the startup costs and figure out how to fill the program more rapidly in order to shorten the period of loss. We calculated that we needed to enroll 120 participants the first year in order to break even. We addressed these issues by constructing a low-income apartment building right next to a PACE day center building. We investigated Housing and Urban Development (HUD)–sponsored low-income housing, but its requirements did not fit our needs. So we decided to raise private funds and build a 120-unit building on our own. Housing would be the attraction; the PACE program would be a nice extra for the residents and would help us fill the program. We could then attract people from local nursing homes to our PACE day center and also offer daytime relief to families who had become overwhelmed by the needs of an increasingly frail parent or spouse living with them.

As we studied PACE programs in order to build our own center, we realized we had not seen a day program actually designed for profoundly frail older adults with special medical and physical needs. Existing adult day programs tended to have developed in church basements or community centers, making do with the space allotted them. They were not suitable for the numbers of clients and the level of assistance that would be required for our PACE participants. Following the pattern of planning and collaboration we had used to design the New Home, we brought in environmental psychologists and architects to design a series of spaces that would facilitate programming for our PACE clients, allow the space to be used for multiple purposes, and encourage collaboration among various care disciplines within the day center's space.

We also realized we hadn't seen any apartment buildings built specifically for profoundly frail older residents. HUD regulations were not focused on supporting design for frailty, but for older people with low incomes. Focusing on frail, poor older adults, and supported by the freedom of having raised our own funds, we were able to build directly for our clients, without having to meet unhelpful regulations dictated by governmental or financing sources. We used ideas we had learned from the New Home and our assisted living buildings, such as short walking distances, wide doorways, and wheelchair-accessible bathrooms. We expected most of our tenants, at least initially, to come to us from nursing homes, and we wanted to be ready for them.

It took 10 years to raise the $12 million we needed to build and open the project. We created 120 unregulated, independent-living apartments designed for frail clients, connected by an enclosed bridge to a PACE health center that would provide the apartment dwellers with services tailored to profoundly frail residents. The center could extend homecare and Meals on Wheels services back to the attached building and into the wider community.

A significant feature of the PACE program was that it co-located participants' frailty caregivers in one place. The engine beginning each day consisted of a multidisciplinary meeting in which everyone involved with a particular client discussed his or her status. Physician, nurse, aide, driver, nutritionist, and physical therapist were all enabled to intervene early and rapidly to head off avoidable declines.

Lessons Learned from PACE

Our PACE experiment had a dramatic impact, but it came at a human and emotional cost. The greatest challenge, and also the greatest opportunity, of the entire exercise was that professionals, clients, families, regulators, and legislators were all required to behave in new ways. The program was new, so it had no history and no local precedents. For the PACE director, there was no experienced guide. Therapists, social workers, and nurses had to work as teams, constantly balancing and negotiating their contributions into a package of wraparound care. Finding people who were willing to try out new ways of caregiving after decades of following standardized routines in hospitals or nursing homes was difficult and exhausting. The director was constantly searching for staff with one hand while negotiating team dynamics with the other.

PACE was just as unfamiliar to the frail clients and their families. There was more independence for older adults—especially for our initial participants who came out of nursing homes to live in our apartments and participate in the PACE program—but they experienced anxiety, as well, as they were called upon to do more for themselves. Families had to engage more than they had when their frail relatives were in nursing homes. Even the most caring family had to feel its way into the new situation.

PACE also created a new dynamic for regulators and the state legislature. When a state decides to venture into a novel approach to healthcare, a new set of ongoing challenges may be set in motion, requiring years of policy discussions. Although the shape and practices of PACE programs are dictated by federal regulations, each state health department may interpret those regulations differently and also execute them differently. The basic tenets of PACE, written into the regulations, have proven very difficult to amend, which dramatically limits the program's ability to serve large numbers of participants. Indeed, health department staff often retain their accustomed nursing home orientation with a single-minded focus on safety and survival. This attitude may lead them to determine that a PACE participant is at too high a risk living outside a nursing home, despite the willingness of the participant and family to take that risk. On the other hand, the state may be fearful that the PACE program will admit participants who are less frail, thereby reaping a financial windfall from the program since those clients' care will be less expensive. Therefore, the state will set the eligibility requirements so high that only extremely frail older adults can be admitted, diminishing the program's opportunities for cost savings by addressing a person's losses earlier in their development.

Some states even leave the responsibility of regulating PACE programs directly to nursing home regulators, but nursing home standards do not always fit PACE programs. A state health department may cap separate sections of a nursing home's reimbursement, for example, allotting a certain amount to nursing, to food, or to management. To apply that scheme to a PACE program deprives it of the flexibility it may need to invest more in management or to change the ratio of physicians to nurses as its clientele changes. Negotiating with various strata of the health department becomes everyday business, critical to the ongoing survival of the nascent PACE program. A newspaper article that brings negative public attention or an oversight in the operation of the PACE program can set in motion a demand for regulatory fixes that almost inevitably have unintended and often far-reaching consequences. PACE administrators must carefully watch the pulse and mood of the legislative and regulatory branches.

Put this all together and it is not surprising to find that the early PACE programs were usually built and sustained by a fiercely committed director who could create all the components of a new paradigm of delivering care while grappling with the community, the legislature, and the state bureaucracy. The work is challenging, full of promise, and very enervating. Even visionary leaders, charged with running such complex and fragile organizations outside the traditional healthcare machine and exposed to waves of change inside the program and out, can't always sustain their energy and vitality. They may burn out before a program matures to sustainability, before the experiment reaches its full potential.

Despite the hurdles built into starting and operating a PACE program, it was an opportunity we couldn't afford to miss. The process taught us a great deal. During its incubation and infancy, the idea, let alone the practice, of government paying for very frail older adults to live outside nursing homes seemed almost incomprehensively dangerous. The concept of deinstitutionalizing very frail people and managing their needs in the community safely and cost-effectively was accompanied by a highly prescriptive program based on the original On Lok model in San Francisco. Because that model was successful, there was an understandable desire for it to be replicated, but it wasn't clear which elements were essential.

PACE programs do continue, nevertheless, and their innovations and successes are legend. But, like the nursing home person-centered care movement established by our New Home, PACE has been overwhelmed by external events. The size, scale, and dimensions of the frailty and aging revolution require systems that are able to expand more rapidly than PACE can. The small scale of its individual programs and its tight regulations, particularly those stipulating highly regimented staff interaction and building-centric approaches to programming, have relegated PACE to the status of a boutique demonstration.

PACE is an experiment that we should keep conducting. It was well worth the effort for us and for our community, but it is not a program that can evolve naturally to meet the needs of an aging nation.

Subsidized Housing

Once we had the PACE Center and its attached 120-unit apartment building open and functioning, we began to look at additional ways we could address the needs of low-income older adults. We turned to government housing, specifically HUD Section 202 Supportive Housing for the Elderly Program. Created by the Housing Act of 1959, the program subsidizes the construction and operation of apartment housing for low-income residents aged 62 and older. In 2016, organizations offering HUD 202 housing were accommodating some 400,000 tenants nationally.[31] My group built three of these subsidized apartment buildings on our campus.

Subsidized housing for low-income seniors was originally conceived as an answer to a very specific housing problem, so it developed in isolation from any other programs addressing aging and required residents to be able to live independently. Congress was anxious to keep programs separate in order to maintain control and financial discipline. Consequently, as residents in HUD 202 apartments aged and began to cope with special needs and incipient frailty, they had no on-site support services or infrastructure. If residents had to use a wheelchair, that might mean the end of subsidized housing for them because their bathroom wasn't accessible. Getting help from an aide would be technically against the building policy that required independence.

Inevitably, residents hid their incipient frailty from the authorities to forestall eviction. The threat of losing an apartment because of frailty was terrifying to someone with few financial resources. Tenants remained secluded in their apartments in fear of having their disabilities discovered. Sometimes groups of tenant vigilantes, in denial of their own future frailty, would watch for and turn in those who acted confused or were bringing in caregivers.

HUD 202 managers originally viewed themselves strictly as rental agents, oblivious to the personal anxieties and needs of the tenants. It was not necessarily due to a lack of sensitivity, but to the dictates of a program designed exclusively for shelter, with absolutely no involvement in healthcare. The entire building was hostage to the narrow concept that we live our lives independently only if we're standing on our own two feet and that we are no longer independent if we need a helping hand. Eventually, HUD came to recognize that aging-in-place was a reality they couldn't ignore. Their program began to provide funds for adapting 202 buildings to frailty as well as for counseling and support services within their walls. If 25% or more of the tenants are frail or at risk of needing specialized care, HUD can now fund a service coordinator to help tenants connect with outside services such as a Medicaid-supported home health aide or Meals on Wheels. HUD may also now give preference to organizations that can build in ways that sustain frailty rather than simply construct and manage real estate.

When the HUD 202 program was started more than 50 years ago, there was no appreciation of how long tenants might live. Policymakers had grown up in a world of considerably lower life expectancy. The assumption was that a resident was independent, and when the person became frail, they would move to a nursing home. Expectations are different today. We now know that many tenants will live into their 80s and 90s, that many will accumulate frailties, and that pushing them out into nursing homes isn't tenable for many reasons, not the least being the reluctance of states to add nursing home costs to their Medicaid budgets.

It has become clear that the addressing the challenges of frail aging adults is not inherently a brick-and-mortar issue but requires programming and supervision as well. We seem to be at the end of the era of stand-alone buildings for older adults. Demographic and economic realities are forcing nursing homes, assisted living facilities, adult homes, and senior housing to integrate with one another. Even so, the size of the coming aging population will be too large to be accommodated in systems based on bricks and mortar, no matter how fast we put up buildings.

Homecare

Before there were nursing homes, everyone aged at home, in the neighborhood where they lived, receiving homecare from relatives. This tradition continues in many communities. These days, people are often discharged from hospitals still needing medical care, so homecare now provides some parts of hospital care, and costs associated with it tend to be an extension of institutional thinking. For example, if a registered nurse comes twice a day for 10 minutes to give a shot, the price must cover the nurse's hourly rate and transportation as well as the medication. Since this is usually less expensive than keeping the client in the hospital, the payer (e.g., insurance company) wants the nurse to see as many outpatients as possible, delivering as many interventions as can be done safely at home. This kind of per-hour or per-procedure approach extends acute care medicine into the community. It generally addresses precise needs for a short duration and does not deal with the ongoing needs of chronic conditions. There is generally little communication between the medical providers and other social services in the community. Even though the care is delivered at home, it does not resemble the kind of coordinated system that we saw around Mrs. Smith in the Introduction.

Along with our other efforts, we developed two different homecare agencies, but because of their restrictive payment systems, we were never able to integrate them with other programs in order to provide more satisfactory continuity of care.

Senior Centers

The Older Americans Act (OAA) was a third, less familiar piece of legislation that accompanied the passage of Medicaid and Medicare in 1965. It called for and initiated community partnerships to serve the social needs of older Americans. The OAA invited local community-based funders to manage social services and programs for older adults.

Under the OAA, small federal outlays are allocated as seed money to stimulate the development of local aging services that are thereafter funded primarily by local dollars. OAA's budget was slightly less than $2.06 billion in 2019, compared with $406 billion for Medicaid. Probably the best-known and most visible example of the OAA community partnership is the local senior center. Communities across the country have constructed and continue to operate buildings that provide social gathering places and a range of activities for older community members. Over time, the OAA added separate funding for complementary services such as transportation and nutrition.

Senior centers in the United States have been an extraordinarily successful movement. All over the nation, the Older Americans Act has stimulated community investment in transportation systems, meal services, and other activities, frequently coordinated by senior centers. Today, 10,000 senior centers serve millions of citizens older than 50 in all 50 states. The centers provide what anthropologists call a third place, after home and work, oriented to the later phase of life. Active seniors shape the centers' activities and programming themselves. As gathering places for relatively healthy seniors, these centers are attractive, and the number of participants is growing.

Yet, the focus on relatively healthy older people limits the senior center's ability to meet the needs of frail men and women living in the community. Frail older adults were never intended to be the senior center's responsibility, and centers have not, for the most part, responded culturally or financially to the large numbers of frail older people suddenly residing nearby. Some have been able to cobble together programs or grants to provide transportation, nutrition, and even some counseling, but their main focus is not on this population.

Often, as members begin to experience losses in personal hygiene and mobility and to show confusion, they are no longer welcome at the senior center, perhaps because they remind their peers of their own vulnerability. Relatively healthy people may filter out the frailer members of the community and cut off people who manifest changes in their physical and mental conditions. The older adults themselves were imprinted by their parents' experiences of aging in an earlier era. The traditional senior center movement, like the original federal low-income housing programs, was designed for independent older adults. These two approaches bookend an old philosophy, both firmly planted in earlier ideas: Independent adults can stay in the community; frail adults must go to an institution.

Senior center staff are typically selected for individual interests and skill sets that fit the primarily independent population. They are not trained for or necessarily comfortable with frailty. The buildings are laid out to address the relatively healthy, ambulatory population that the OAA legislation anticipated decades ago. New senior centers are still being built around that very focused conceptualization, locked into serving only a particular slice of seniors by dint of the design of the original federal program as well a decades-long culture.

The OAA and its senior centers are now experiencing the massive entrance of Boomer seniors, who will undoubtedly re-create senior centers in their own image. But there is no reason to believe that the centers will attempt to adapt their resources to frail older adults living in the community or to integrate these people into their midst.

When a large regional senior center needed to vacate their building, we had preliminary discussions about the possibility of relocating them to our property. Negotiations never proceeded, however, in large measure because the senior center served independent older adults, which was programmatically distinct from our initiatives to address frail older people.

The Disconnect between Medical and Community Programs

In 2008, I participated in an 18-month fellowship sponsored by a Buffalo foundation focused on improving outcomes for vulnerable populations. Individuals were arranged in small teams of five or six. My group included executives from our two major hospital systems, the CEO of a health-oriented foundation, and the director of the region's largest senior center. Our team studied the problem of how to transfer frail older adults from hospitals back to their homes safely. Our initial working assumption was that the interaction between the hospital system and the community system was not properly managed and that, with better communication and coordination, transfers could be conducted in an acceptable manner.

We convened a meeting of discharge planners from the major hospitals. It took a few moments for them to become comfortable talking to us, and then the floodgates opened. They were under enormous pressure from the hospitals to discharge frail older patients, but they explained that there were minimal community resources to help with the transition. By and large, the traditional agencies were not responsive. It took weeks to arrange for Meals on Wheels for a discharging client, for example, or for other agencies to determine if a person was appropriate for services that were geared for relatively well and stable older adults.

From the point of view of the hospital discharge planners, the community services responded too slowly and had no capacity to coordinate their programs with other necessary services. Our original hypothesis had been wrong. The reality was not that the hospital and community gears did not mesh, but rather that there were no effective community gears at all. The discharge planners asked if we could help develop the programs they needed to integrate frail older adults back into their homes and neighborhoods. Our team was not in a position to be much help at the time, but I never forgot their dilemma.

Disaster Reveals the Nature of the Frailty Challenge

Early in October 2006, the Buffalo area was hit with an early freak snowstorm that piled 2 feet of snow on the region. Accustomed to long, snowy winters, most Western New Yorkers would not normally have blinked an eye at such an event in December or January. But this particular unexpected tempest blew in while the trees were still covered with leaves. As the snow accumulated, its weight on leafy branches felled trees that had survived decades of squalls and blizzards. Power lines were disrupted throughout the region as falling trees and heavy ice knocked them down. Electricity went out for over a week in more than 300,000 households, and many roads were so choked with fallen trees that repairs were not completed for many days.

Debris, twisted limbs, and live wires were strewn everywhere, making it impossible to drive on many streets even after the snow had melted. Most Western New Yorkers were stranded. The routines of everyday life became impossible in a region famous for handling inclement weather. For many, the disruption was an unusually annoying inconvenience, and hardy Buffalonians lit their living rooms by candle and relied on stored supplies of soup for dinner. Many even learned to entertain themselves without the benefit of a television screen.

Sometimes neighbors were able to help each other, but as the authorities went door to door, checking to make sure families were equipped to survive, they found a segment of Western New Yorkers in perilous straits. In houses and apartments throughout the region they discovered hundreds of older adults, many frightened beyond their wits, confused, frail, and hungry. They were stranded with nowhere to turn for help. Most were scooped up and deposited at whichever hospitals and nursing homes had the capacity to provide a cot and some warmth and food. At our facility, they trickled in, with a police cruiser stopping by to walk a few blanket-wrapped men and women into the lobby. Then, as the days passed, they just kept coming. Before long, facilities throughout the region were inundated. For those who care for the region's older adults, it was a "Katrina Moment." The natural disaster suddenly shed light on a portion of the community that had been frequently forgotten: old, frail Buffalonians living at home alone, largely hidden away from the rest of the world.

We had known there were people living in the community with profiles similar to those in nursing homes, but when the storm hit and people started arriving at our door, we were shocked by their numbers and the scale of their needs. It took me a while to realize how extreme their circumstances were. They were living without any safety net, in fragile circumstances, and at great risk, especially when compared to the robust systems, crosschecks, and resources with which I was familiar in a nursing home. We were accustomed to feeding, clothing, ambulating, toileting, and medicating our residents, no matter how frail or poor or alone they were. As we put our own residents in their clean, dry beds, it dawned on us very slowly what the storm was showing us. The scene made me recall time I had spent in Calcutta in 1971. I stayed in a Salvation Army hostel, and each morning when I departed, I was instantly surrounded by dozens of men, women, and children living on the street in absolute squalor, with arms outstretched begging for money. They were so small and emaciated that I could clear myself a path with a gentle sweep of my arm.

The quiet, frail, desperate older adults disgorged by the October snowstorm awakened that memory. I suddenly understood the desperate plight of frail older people living invisibly in my own community. Over the decades of my working experience, supports for complex, long-term care for the frail population had mutated. Too many needy people, I realized, had fallen off the grid. They were the ones who didn't qualify for nursing homes, couldn't afford assisted living, and didn't know how to access any other parts of the care system for aging. They remained where they had lived in their earlier years, despite their changed physical, emotional, cognitive, and financial circumstances, stranded in an environment that had become alien and with no one to help them.

Some had the well-intentioned support of relatives, but the situations of frail people who remain in their homes tend to be frustrating both for them and for their family members. The problems keep changing and can be hard to identify. Families may have few resources of their own and often no connections to a healthcare system or community agencies. Because society could no longer increase the supply of facilities to house them, these frail older adults were left with no alternative but lonely and dangerous isolation in the community.

Formulating a Plan

How could we help this group? Through our own efforts, we had already become aware that widespread placement in nursing homes was not feasible, assisted living was unaffordable, senior housing was scarce and often not sufficiently supportive, and existing homecare was inadequate. PACE programs were not capable of expanding to the scale of the aging population, and senior centers were for those who were still healthy. What was needed, we believed, was a brand-new concept: a place where older adults could have access to the integrated care of a nursing home but sleep in their own beds rather than require the government to house them. It seemed to us that there were resources available that could be combined to do the job, but they were distributed throughout various disconnected programs and agencies. If we could link them together, perhaps we could create a support system for profoundly frail community members who were living outside of nursing homes.

We resolved to try to co-locate as many existing community programs and resources as possible in a single building. We were not encouraging the organizations to merge, but simply to install themselves next to one another. The logic for grouping them was clear to us. Many small community agencies such as Catholic Charities, Jewish Family Services, dementia day services, food pantries, and geriatric medical clinics were at risk because of reductions in government and private support. Each had thrived earlier when government grants were available, when their boards were filled with businesspeople who raised and donated money for them, and when staffing had been relatively inexpensive.

By the early 21st century, everything had changed. The business leaders who created and supported the nonprofit organizations no longer provided help because the government had replaced them. Then, governments reduced financial support, and local foundations became overwhelmed with requests. Historic, specialized community agencies found themselves struggling. At the same time, since many frail older adults were no longer scooped up and out of the community and into nursing homes, the community agencies were being asked to serve a greater number of clients, many with more chronic and serious conditions than they were accustomed to handling. Their staff members were constantly frustrated by the complexity of their clients' needs and their agencies' inability to coordinate interventions that would help. As caring people, they were deflated and depressed. We wanted to offer them an opportunity to extend their reach and regain their footing in the community by opening satellite offices in our center.

This was surprisingly difficult. During the Industrial Age, agency executives had been encouraged to become competitive with other nonprofits for increasingly limited grants and donors. Even though leading organizations like the United Way had been attempting to merge community agencies, it was usually an impossible challenge. The first priority of a CEO was to assure the survival of his or her own agency, a corollary of which was to maintain his or her position. We met with these fiercely independent agency executives individually to share with them our discovery of the tragically frail segment of society that had been brought into our nursing home after the October storm. With profoundly frail older adults living in the community as our focus, we pointed out that none of us alone could manage the care that was required for them, as every executive was aware. We told them that the new organization that we were planning, which we called the Town Square for Aging, was not centrally controlled but was conceived to be a true collaboration among agencies. Each agency would have its own space and would control its own operation in the building. The new factor would be the building itself, which would house them all in one location.

We raised millions of dollars to refit a building, allowing each agency to fashion a space appropriate for its operational needs. We spent years meeting, discussing, sharing, and uncovering potential synergies. Our idea was that older men and women would arrive at the Town Square for Aging when they needed help in getting their lives to run smoothly and safely. We expected that they would come in at first for a single reason—to visit a pharmacy, food bank, or hairdresser—but that the first contact would only be a beginning. The real innovation in care would come as each agency gathered information from them and then engaged other co-located programs to address other problems as they were revealed. The proximity of providers in the Town Square would make this possible, by making it easy for the older adult, after picking up his or her prescription or getting a haircut, to walk down the hall to talk to a physical therapist, tax preparer, or nurse.

Simply co-locating agencies, of course, is not sufficient for providing truly integrated services. But by listening, analyzing, and then walking with the client to the next resource for help, the Town Square for Aging sought to develop a cumulative and multifaceted approach to the varied and interacting challenges confronting the client and his or her family. We imagined that as we learned more about a client, a new provider would move to center stage momentarily. The new provider would have the advantage of cumulative knowledge about why the client had come to the Town Square and what additional services were needed. Each agency would consider how to integrate new help with what was already being provided. When something gave way in the complex of variables that held the client in equilibrium, as happens periodically, the Town Square members could be there for a rethinking and perhaps a recalibration. The family would have a caring location where their family member could network and find support. The co-location of services in the Town Square for Aging would also foster informal interactions between the agencies that would enable them to work together to the benefit of the aged clients.

We knew that thousands of profoundly frail older adults were isolated and inadequately served. They and their families were so dispersed and overwhelmed that, despite their need, they were in no position themselves to help us organize or disseminate information. Their plight was so raw and immediate that we were careful not to go public until we were completely up and running, for fear of experiencing an immediate avalanche of requests for help or of cruelly arousing expectations that we couldn't yet meet.

Limitations of Co-locating Existing Community Programs

The need for integrated care was great and was increasing every day as fewer older adults were finding suitable places in facilities. The co-location plan was logical and compelling. The participating agency executives were all well intentioned, but even after years of collaborative energy, the Town Square for Aging was never fully realized.

While the benefits to frail clients seemed clear, the benefits to the organizations themselves were not as obvious. There was no mechanism for passing back to the Town Square or its participants any of the savings from reducing hospitalizations or unnecessary health costs. The CEOs of the participating agencies did not know one another well. Even if they saw some potential benefits to their own organizations from having a place in the Town Square, it was hard for them to think in terms of the larger group that was gathered. Their responses would often rebound back to loyalty to their individual agencies. The divisions between agencies that had developed during the highpoint of the Industrial Age in the 1950s remained firmly in place, even though this meant that they were unable to meet the more complex needs of the population in the community.

The Town Square organizations were also daunted by the task of learning to coordinate with one another. Almost everyone recognized that it was critically important to share information. Starting with the idea that a client should not have to replicate basic background data as he or she moved among the providers in the building, we began to think about how to create a shared log of a client's various evaluations and the interventions that had been used. Along the way, we recognized that each agency had no easy way to understand what others were doing. We all used very different features of Medicaid, Medicare, and other programs, and each group had developed its own ways to navigate the system. We were swimming in a chaotic thicket of data, with little ability to make sense of it for clients or for ourselves. Our hope was that over time, with the anticipated intimacy provided by the co-location, we would slowly become more comfortable sharing information and would develop digital approaches to sharing. That collaboration never had a chance to develop.

The large nonprofit-managed healthcare organization that had renovated a large medical suite in the building was unable to find appropriate practitioners to provide the medical staff they needed, and then their own unrelated financial difficulties dissuaded their leadership from investing in a new venture. Without the presence of a large managed care organization to bring clients into the Town

Square, there was little confidence that the new setup could garner community support quickly enough.

The hospitals, community physicians, and large service organizations, all of which could have sent us clients that were of no financial benefit to them, chose not to engage. They tended to see the Town Square effort either as inconsequential and not worthy of their time, or as a potential threat to their control of the client within the old medical paradigm. Even though it was based in part in the familiar business concept of co-location of space—using centrality to extend services—it could not garner the engagement of the existing healthcare players, who remained in their historic traditional roles. Healthcare leadership was unalterably institution bound.

The Town Square concept required that everyone involved take enormous risks into new behaviors, relationships, and constructs while continuing to maintain ongoing responsibilities to their survival in their current paradigm. It was an attempt to knit together elements of the existing landscape to create something new and more effective. It required leaps from the existing paradigm that were dramatic and required an allocation of resources that was not yet imaginable. In the end, it was too different from the traditional methods of care delivery for the organizations, the individual clients, and even the community at large to engage. Looking back, perhaps we were too ambitious. Or perhaps we were not ambitious enough.

Conclusion

The difficulties that we encountered in trying to launch the Town Square for Aging strengthened our earlier realizations that none of the available options for aging care would be adequate for the size of the upcoming population of frail individuals. We realized that no solution existed for this massive societal shift. This is still true today. Even the language that we commonly use in discussing the field no longer captures the underlying realities. Our so-called *continuum of care*, for example, is not continuous. It excludes major services from its program, forcing people to jump on and off the continuum as their needs change. *Levels of care* are more inconsistent than they are level because each tier expands and contracts according to changes in reimbursement. A single level often contains a cohort of clients with profiles that seem to belong to levels that were historically above or below it. An experience of *long-term care* may actually be composed of a series of short-term situations. The word *disease* is misleading because it suggests phenomena from the world of acute care that are very different from the chronic conditions that older adults experience. *Nursing home* is as outdated a term as its predecessor, *rest homes*, for the emphasis in these institutions has shifted from traditional nursing care to therapies and medical interventions, and anyway, they rarely feel like home. *Independent living* suggests absolute independence, a particularly pernicious idea when in fact every resident lives with some amount of assistance. *Assisted living* attaches the need for assistance to the older person's physical abode and may impact his or her self-image. *Homecare* carries with it notions of isolation and a thin patina of intermittent services. Much of our language contains connotations that are simply inaccurate or pejorative.

Many of these words act as dividers, isolating older people from the rest of us. It's difficult to find one's way, even to discuss the possibilities, when the words commonly used have meanings that do not capture the underlying realities. New language is needed to convey the dynamics of a new world and to focus on an individual's attributes and needs, rather than a category based on a person's location.

The new world of aging should not be seen as a group of microcosms to be addressed solely within narrow professional areas, such as long-term care management or legal strategies for intergenerational wealth management. It's a new condition for all of society.

After all of our efforts, we realized it was time to rethink the care for our aging cohort in the United States.

PART II

What Is Really Happening

CHAPTER 8

Chronic Conditions and Benescence

The New State of Well-Being in Older Age

At some point in developing the narrowly targeted care programs for older adults described previously, I had to sit back and wonder where we were going wrong. We had built a new style of nursing home that worked the way we thought it should. We had followed that achievement with assisted living facilities of more than one type, low-income senior housing, an innovative PACE program, adult day services, homecare, and finally the Town Square for Aging. We were racing faster and faster, but the needs we wanted to meet seemed to be racing ahead of us. Why wouldn't the pieces fall into place the way we wanted?

After 30 years of attempting to build, adapt, and innovate robust appropriate systems to meet the new aging imperative, I had failed to find a system that would work in today's world with its enormous number of older adults, many of them becoming frail and living with their frailty for many years. Each of the aging programs we developed seemed to have its own internally designed limits, in addition to being repeatedly stifled by the difficulties of overcoming the complex regulations and the silos of bureaucracy. The aging care system as a whole was like a tree covered with ivy so thick and lush that it girdled the tree's trunk and covered all its limbs. Eventually the thick vines of regulations, court precedents, tight administrative scrutiny, and protectionism within the industry itself strangled the system. Green shoots of restrictions and barricades quickly covered each spurt of growth. The branches and leaves could no longer reach for the sun, and the entity failed to thrive.

What were we missing as we tried to break through this tangled web? Could it be something so fundamental that it never came to mind? There is an old Gary Larson cartoon in which two cowboys are riding along the range and one rears back and says, "Whoa, we forgot the cattle!" I came to realize that along the way, our efforts had missed the heart of the matter. The real issue is not getting older in years, but the phenomenon of chronic conditions. Furthermore, the word "disease," when it is associated with older adults, has an entirely different meaning from the one we normally give it. No wonder I had arrived without the cattle!

Living in the Age of Extended Chronic Conditions

Our cultural understanding of the nature of disease is still based on the belief that acute disease is the fundamental culprit that affects most lives. Until around 100 years ago, widespread infectious diseases like smallpox or tuberculosis that could kill people at any age were the primary threat to human health. Today, however, that element, which held true through all the previous millennia of human existence, is no longer dominant. Even the horrific COVID-19 pandemic is responsible for a relatively small percentage of the annual death rate. In the United States, of the 3,458,697 deaths in 2021, approximately 460,000 involved COVID-19 as the underlying cause or contributing cause.[32] COVID constituted only 13.2% of annual mortality in the United States, including many of the frail older adults who already had pre-existing chronic conditions and perhaps a very limited life expectancy.*

One of the defining conditions of our current existence is our new ability to stave off death, often for years. Infectious and other deadly diseases have been succeeded in importance and widespread impact by degenerative diseases such as cardiovascular problems, cancer, or arthritis, conditions that do not kill in a short time and that we can live with into older age. Even widespread pandemics can eventually be brought under control. We have redirected what seemed previously to be one of the fundamental conditions of life by changing the face of illness. But we haven't yet sufficiently changed our attitudes and fears about disease to match this new reality.

As I have already described, when the Baby Boomers were born in the middle of the 20th century, medicine seemed able to achieve

---

*Note that the ballyhooed 1 million U.S. COVID deaths is a cumulative total over multiple years. None of this is to dismiss or diminish the pain and tragedy of the COVID-19 epidemic. Rather, it attempts to place it in a fuller historical epidemiologic context.

almost anything, as perhaps most strikingly exemplified by the polio vaccines. Sickness had always threatened life, but now medicine was powerful enough to threaten sickness. Hospitals were fitted with dozens of new ways to cure people, and medical research labs were filled with the smartest people who had ever lived. Medicine and public health found ways to protect us from many potentially fatal diseases. And if we can't vanquish a disease outright, we can often turn an absolute killer into a chronic condition, as we did with HIV/AIDS, or reduce its morbidity, as the COVID vaccines have done.

Medicine has not conquered all infectious disease, as the COVID-19 virus has shown us. We still get sick, and we still die, even though we spend more on our health than we ever have before. Yet, the balance has changed. The landscape has a new form. Today, barring rare emergencies like the pandemic, and unlike the mid-20th century, most people who are sick are old, and most of what ails them are chronic conditions. This shift, like the growth of the numbers of the older population, is still so recent that we don't fully realize we're living in it. When we think of medicine, we still tend to envision variations on the basic television medical drama storyline: Find the problem, save the patient. But that's not what most healthcare is actually like today. Unlike acute disease, illness in late life often comes to stay, and illnesses pile up. People in their 80s have bodies that are less resilient but that nonetheless continue to function. Older adults live many years with illnesses that probably would have killed our ancestors if they hadn't succumbed to an infectious disease much sooner. We get sick and, thanks to medicine and the healthy start we now get, we live on.

In the early 20th century, when infectious diseases were the biggest killers, older men and women were also burdened with chronic conditions, but they didn't live as long, and there was not much to do for them, so they didn't incur as much expense. We are now living decades longer than we did 100 years ago, and there are many more of us. In 2050, when the youngest of the Baby Boomers will be 86, we will have a different, older nation. Social Security and Medicare will be providing resources for many more years of life than their designers anticipated.

Compromising chronic conditions have long been considered an inevitable part of being old. The fact that these conditions may be avoided or dramatically mitigated in our later years is only just beginning to be understood and has not sunk into the general consciousness. As I mentioned previously, we are now experiencing an Age of Extended Chronic Conditions.

When we get a degenerative disease, such as arthritis, medicine stabilizes and then maintains us. If we get another degenerative disease, perhaps glaucoma, medicine stabilizes and then maintains us on that front; then another, if necessary, and another. We can live with multiple chronic conditions. Carefully balancing conditions and adapting treatments maintains our health. This is entirely different from the treatment of acute diseases, which often go away or are cured by short-term treatment, rather than being managed over long periods.[+]

Chronic conditions may arise at any age, but when they occur later in life, the years may have made the body less efficient and used up much of its once-abundant reserves. One of our organs may start to misfire, followed by another. We tune ourselves up with medication and maybe some surgery along the way. As we get deep into very old age, our health may depend on a mix of several interventions. Managing multiple chronic conditions late in life is a compound, multidimensional problem.

Dealing with Chronic Conditions

The nature of what we commonly call chronic conditions challenges the way we define disease. If you can manage a condition such as rheumatoid arthritis with medication so that the symptoms disappear, do you still have the condition? You are not ill in the sense that it is usually meant. When you have chest pain that sends you to your cardiologist, who then sends you to the hospital to have a defibrillator or a pacemaker implanted, are you less healthy when you get home the next day than you were the day before? When exactly were you "diseased" in this chain of events?[33,34] Having a chronic condition or

---

[+]There are exceptions and overlapping conditions. For example, we are discovering that even if someone is cured of a COVID-19 infection, there may be long-term chronic conditions that the individual will have to live with. Many of the people who developed polio in the 1950s and were thought to have recovered fully are in their later years showing symptoms that can be traced back to the original illness.

two is not really being ill or diseased as we normally use the terms. At the onset of a chronic condition, you may be aware of limitations, but medication or a change in diet or physical therapy can often return you to something approximating your previous functional status.

The World Health Organization prefers to think about defining disability and its impact on activities of daily living (ADLs) or instrumental activities of daily living (IADLS)‡ rather than using the term "disease." If you have otosclerosis that impacts your hearing and you get a hearing aid, you have a hearing impairment when the hearing aids are not working. A cardiac pacemaker keeps your heart beating at the right rate, but if its battery fails you still have the underlying cardiac condition.

We have tended to think of health and illness as a kind of binary state. You are healthy and you don't need healthcare or you are unhealthy and you do need healthcare. A chronic condition doesn't belong on either side of this equation, however. It is a continuing process, during which the need for healthcare may vary, and it plays some role in the lives of most 80- to 100-year-olds. Our joints function differently, as do our digestive system, skin, and sensory organs. We begin to avoid stairs and spicy food, we add sunscreen, sunglasses, and hearing aids. We accommodate to an altered state of being for chronic conditions, but we do not necessarily consider ourselves sick.

Chronic conditions can be hard to see from the outside, which makes it harder for those who have not yet experienced them to understand. The developed world appears to be filled with healthy people, but a considerable number of them, mostly older adults, are actually living with chronic conditions and receiving healthcare to manage them. Many of us do not count these people among the sick, even if we are aware of their conditions.

Because we haven't adjusted our thinking to acknowledge the shift from the time when most healthcare was for acute diseases to the present when chronic conditions predominate, we don't yet care for the older members of our society as well as we could. Our care systems, which are still oriented to treating acute disease, are not

---

‡IADLs are not necessary for fundamental functioning, but they let an individual live independently in a community.

set up for the needs of older people who are sometimes frail with chronic problems. In order to care for them appropriately, we first need to understand that their conditions are caused by chronic conditions and not simply by being older.

Chronic conditions in older age need to be addressed as a healthcare issue separate from old age itself. When people talk about aging, the conversation, either at the kitchen table or as part of the national discourse, is often framed in terms of resources. It is usually an anxious discussion. What happens when the money runs out? Will the national economy survive the coming avalanche of aging Baby Boomers? Are we saving enough for our later years? Yet, chronic conditions in old age actually underlie these worries. For some fortunate older adults, the house is paid for, the children are no longer dependent, the wardrobe is simpler, travel is less ambitious, and the pace is less hectic. Many others with fixed or insufficient income may have trouble meeting housing and food costs. For many of us, however, healthcare costs will bring us to a moment when we run out of money and there is no obvious way out.

Although healthcare costs are certainly an area of great financial concern for older adults (frequently a health event tips over the precarious financial balance), it is, paradoxically, aging itself that is blamed for the crisis. This is not correct. The phenomenon of aging—the greater number of years in and of themselves—isn't the problem. Rather, chronic conditions are the problem. It's like the second impact in a car crash. The first impact (age) is the car hitting the tree, but the second impact (chronic conditions) is the driver hitting the inside of the car. Historically, manufacturers developed bumpers and other car protections for the inevitable accidents on the road. However, manufacturers did not install seatbelts and airbags until Ralph Nader[35] insisted that the impact on people in the interior of the car was a correlated and perhaps even more critical consequence of vehicular accidents.

Illness in older adults may be correlated with their advanced years, but it is not directly caused by it any more than mononucleosis is caused by adolescence. Until fairly recently, it was accepted that mental deterioration late in life was an inevitable function of aging. We called it senility. Many kinds of dementia, like Alzheimer's disease, do occur most often later in life, but they are caused by changes in the brain or sensory limitations, not by the number of years someone has lived.[§] If we understand Alzheimer's disease as an illness rather than an unavoidable development, we will realize that we can work on its prevention and management and perhaps even find a cure. The same holds for many of the maladies correlated with older age that have not yet received sufficient attention.

If a disease associated with aging occurred with the same frequency in younger people, we would not think of it as a problem largely associated with their age cohort, but as a disease problem. We would worry about the costs associated with the disease, not about the costs associated with being a particular age. Separating old age from the incidence of illness in old age may seem like splitting hairs, but it's not a fine point. It's a distinction that is fundamental to figuring out how we can develop into a society that helps us live comfortably as we live longer and longer.

Well-Being in Older Age: The State of Benescence

We sometimes call the process of getting older "senescence," a negatively charged word that refers to all the losses and deteriorations that come as the years go by. The term is a telling example of how we see older age using primarily negative terms. If we understand that chronic conditions are not disease in the traditional sense, however, we can come to a deeper understanding of health in our later years and posit what we might call a State of Benescence (a combination of "bene" meaning well or good and "senescence" meaning old age). This may occur when the process of aging can include a sense of well-being, derived from the effective management of chronic conditions, from the benefits of experience and accumulated understanding, and from the pleasures of having a role in the community. The concept of a State of Benescence provides a new model for understanding health in older age. In this model, even people with multiple chronic conditions can qualify as being in a State of Benescence, rather than sick.

Over time, as we all know, every organ and system in the body changes. A 1-year-old is incontinent, has trouble walking, and has

---

§ Increased age does increase the risk of Alzheimer's disease because there has been more time for beta amyloid to build up in the brain. Perhaps it is more accurate to say that years of life is not a proximate causation or correlation, but a distal one.

minimal judgment, but for his or her age the child is in a state of well-being. We buy diapers, baby-proof the house, substitute our judgment for his or hers, and think the child is doing just fine. Perhaps the same evaluation can be applied to a 102-year-old with chronic conditions, and we can consider the person to be in a State of Benescence and doing just fine at his or her age.

We often equate health with the most perfect state the body can achieve. Such perfection would have to include, for example, the number and strength of a 10-year-old's taste buds and a 20-year-old's sexual energy. The image of perfect health would be the Classical Greek athlete or goddess, thereby making the rest of our 80-plus years nothing but a slow deterioration. Do we really wish to define the human lifespan that way? Is all life after 20 a period of deterioration? Or is there a more generous definition of healthiness, one that's more inclusive and that describes our actual life experience?

Our bodies and our minds don't start changing when we get to old age. They have been changing all along. Children transform dramatically as they grow; older adults change in appearance almost as dramatically as they grow older. We shed, we swap new cells for old, we grow, we shrink, and we gain and lose muscle mass. Each period of our lives has its version of a State of Benescence.

This idea of a State of Benescence does not include believing that nothing can be done for a 102-year-old, nor does it suggest that the older person should be resigned to his or her various chronic conditions. That would be as cruel as not treating diaper rash at age 1, acne at age 13, or eyesight changes at age 40. As at any age, our goal should be to prevent diseases when we can and to minimize their adverse consequences when we can't eliminate them completely. We should alleviate the effects of the chronic conditions that have piled up in the 102-year-old body as much as possible, reducing pain and increasing mobility. This provides the older adult with a quality of life that he or she finds acceptable, so that the person considers him- or herself to be in a State of Benescence. It's a new state from earlier periods in his or her life, but it's okay nonetheless—and an improvement over how the person felt before interventions were introduced. The fact that chronic conditions arise does not mean that an older adult cannot be helped to a State of Benescence.

Seeing a State of Benescence as a desired condition shifts us away from the acute disease framework that often has insufficient approaches for those with chronic issues. The concept of a state of well-being suggests a positive approach to the whole person that uses everything available, from medication, to helping hands, to small devices around the house that all maintain the State of Benescence. We marshal our assets as best we can to live as well as we can. We adjust and adapt in order to remain in a State of Benescence, but we aren't getting cured in the sense of having a particular condition go completely away. We are no longer necessarily going to outgrow the diagnoses we receive. In past times, older people simply endured the chronic conditions that were felt to be inseparable from getting old. Now we push back, demand interventions, and aspire to rebalance or recalibrate our State of Benescence. We haven't thrown off the chronic condition, but we have learned to mitigate its effects in significant ways. The hope, which I address later, is that we develop a delivery system that will extend appropriate approaches to everyone, not just those in higher socio-economic groups.

The 75- to 80-year-olds in the locker room at the golf club in Sunny Haven, SC, where they have migrated in their retirement, are knobby folks who won't be mistaken for 50-year-olds and who no longer exude much athleticism, but they are lacing up their golf shoes to play. They are likely to have impressively long medical resumes, including bypass surgery, blood thinners, beta blockers, persistent heartburn, glaucoma, hearing aids, pacemakers, blood pressure pills, and other kinds of support. They may not look hardy, but they're still pretty hale. A generation or two ago, many at that chronological age with the same underlying conditions would have been in rocking chairs with rugs on their laps. A generation or two before that, most would have been dead.

Acute and Chronic Care

Perhaps surprisingly, this conversation about tuning and balancing chronic conditions in older age is a new one. We don't yet have a widely shared understanding of the new state of chronicity. Even for older adults themselves as they go through their changes, the notion that it is possible to arrive at an advanced age, have a combination of chronic conditions, and still be in a State of Benescence is not yet easy to accept, or to see as being as common as it is. Many people still conflate aging with the chronic conditions that people incur late in life, and they find it impossible to see the person apart from his or her conditions. That confusion of aging with chronic conditions has led to the common but mistaken assumption that advanced age causes chronic conditions and that living with chronic conditions prevents a person from a State of Benescence. This is not a harmless misunderstanding.

Conclusion

Older adults are not sick with age any more than children are sick with being young. We don't have to cure age itself. To confuse the chronic conditions that are more prevalent in old age with aging itself is to conflate a stage of life with disease. Sadly, the confusion often means that older people suffer much more than they need to because intervening is not considered worthwhile. It takes a determined effort to change one's thinking and separate the conditions from older age, but the effort is worth the new understanding it provides: that our later years are not something to fear in and of themselves. In other words, one can be in a State of Benescence in older age. We continue to find ways to accommodate chronic conditions and physical limitations, but because we still habitually mix up older age and chronic conditions, we can't see chronic conditions as clearly as we need to. We cannot appreciate their complexities or see how plastic and malleable they may be. We don't perceive how our deepening understanding of chronic conditions is speeding up our ability to manage them so that very old age can still be a State of Benescence.

CHAPTER 9

Delivering and Paying for the State of Benescence

Care for older adults accounts for a lion's share of our healthcare spending. The system's ingrained practices are unfortunately not designed to address the chronic problems that we live with today. We have enjoyed the benefits of amazing medical breakthroughs in recent decades, but the way we deliver our care hasn't changed to reflect the advances. Our hospital infrastructure is a legacy from the days when acute diseases ruled. It collects the sick in order to treat them together and efficiently. Clients recover and go home, but as chronic conditions have superseded acute disease, this model has become outdated. As a result, one of the principal reasons for the continuing existence of the traditional hospital design has shrunk dramatically. Even though we live in a world of chronic conditions, we receive care in a world of acute disease that does not have the systems or knowledge to care for chronic conditions, especially the multiple ones of the expanding frail older population. We distort our approach to chronic conditions when we call them diseases, a term that implies they can be cured and disappear. We can't adequately address the chronic world from the acute one because we don't cure a chronic condition. We ameliorate and manage it across an extended lifespan.

Delivering Healthcare

The current relationship between acute and chronic care is anything but benign. The medical establishment, mostly dedicated to the acute care model, jealously guards its dominance by robbing chronic care of resources and viability. The costs of acute medicine leave few residual resources or energy for long-term interventions that prevent the exacerbation of chronic conditions and the eventual need for medical interventions. It's a self-reinforcing, closed-loop system. Resources are reserved only for the most dire and dramatic situations.

Less pressing chronic conditions are not deemed worthy of attention until they mature to require acute care. The hegemony of acute care so shapes the healthcare culture that alternatives are not funded or pursued to any significant extent, crippling the development of chronic care. The focus on acute needs limits our attention, for example, to developing methods for heading off disasters such as metabolic syndrome, a cluster of conditions that increase the risk of heart disease, stroke, and diabetes. Many of the 3 million new cases of this syndrome each year could be handled through long-term preventive measures, but under the current regime they are seriously addressed only when they ripen and become worthy of medical specialty care.

For the person who needs nonurgent chronic care and health maintenance, the kind of singular fix that dominates procedure-based hospital care is often insufficient. Instead, an intervention that resolves one problem must be considered in the context of other interventions. So, the client can no longer be the "heart attack in room 233" or the "appendectomy in room 401," but rather the dehydrated 95-year-old in room 305 with diabetes, chronic kidney disease, macular degeneration, and nascent depression, all of which must be considered with each new step in treatment. It is often an impossible challenge to the traditional hospital to coordinate and accommodate the recommendations of various separate, procedure-focused professionals so that they reach the optimal outcome.

Usually, and very unfortunately, the older adult gets lost in the highly specialized environment of the modern hospital. The presenting problem, whether a broken hip or pneumonia, is the one that is addressed. Other conditions are set aside, even when this is harmful to the patient. There is no delivery platform in the hospital as it is configured today that can carefully and attentively administer the range of interventions necessary for a frail older person with compounding problems. It actually becomes urgent to get the person out of the hospital because his or her unattended underlying conditions begin to worsen and require treatment that will not be reimbursed.

For many years, by both plan and inertia, state health departments and the federal government have retarded the updating of our care delivery system. A relatively benign interpretation might be that even though they were aware that specific procedures could be delivered by lower, less costly interventions, policymakers were loath to

disturb the fragile financial condition of hospitals by allowing procedures to be replaced in less expensive settings. They were cognizant
that hospitals need to retain control over the greatest possible array
of services in order to remain solvent and that there has been only
a thin layer of government funding available for frail older adults. A
less benign interpretation is the suspicion that policymakers were
either oblivious to the problems or were in the thrall of the powerful hospitals. In either case, this stance is no longer in line with the
needs of the current population in the United States. Although only
17% of Americans are over 65, people of that age group constitute
almost 40% of hospitalized adults, and many of them have chronic
conditions that need attention.[36]

We need to develop a new understanding of the care needs of
our older citizens in order to serve them properly. Once we redefine
care as it relates to older age, in particular recognizing the defining
role of chronic conditions, we will understand more precisely why
the current system for care delivery does not work for our oldest citizens. We must consider caring for people outside of hospitals and
medical offices as well as within them. More older adults are living
longer with chronic conditions, and they are desperate for an overall
system that responds to their continuing needs in a coordinated way
that they can understand.

The story of the medical specialty of geriatrics in the United
States illustrates the problem. Late in the 20th century, it was hoped
that geriatrics, a new field, would provide multidisciplinary leadership in the coming wave of chronic conditions. However, the under-
funding of geriatricians has hobbled the expected development of the
field. The complexity of diagnosis of older clients and the weighing
and balancing of all their accumulating interventions make geriatrics
unappealing and unremunerative in the existing acute healthcare
system.* In outpatient medical offices financial viability is based on
volume and speed, but older clients require more time for diagnosis
and are slower to move through their appointments. As a result, the

---

* In 2019 rankings of salaries by healthcare specialty, family medicine was listed #18 out
of 20, right above certified registered nurse anesthetist and nurse practitioner (geriatrics was
not listed). (Physician starting salaries by specialty: 2019 vs 2018. Merritt Hawkins, August 6,
2019, https://www.merritthawkins.com/news-and-insights/blog/healthcare-news-and-trends/
physician-starting-salaries-by-specialty-2019-vs-2018/.)

numbers of geriatric-focused outpatient venues are inadequate. As I will explain later, nursing homes are evolving into more acute and short-term centers, and geriatricians are losing their roles as coordinators even in the domains where their expertise has historically been critical. At a time when such competence can be invaluable, too few venues exist for optimizing their skill sets. As a result, trained and experienced geriatricians can be scarce.[†]

The fact that healthcare for older adults, especially in hospitals, is based on an outdated model parallels what we have also seen to be true of the existing options for long-term aging. The system is even forcing nursing homes, historically the last refuge in the United States for frail adults, to focus on acute problems, leaving those with chronic conditions in the lurch. The reimbursement systems that fund nursing homes increasingly favor short-term, acute interventions. Many states face budget shortfalls, so they are reducing their Medicaid reimbursements, forcing nursing homes to turn to federally funded Medicare. Because Medicare is focused on short-term care, nursing homes are increasingly dependent on filling beds with short-term clients undergoing aggressive interventions, giving them a greater resemblance to hospitals than to traditional institutions of long-term care. Care protocols become dominated by hospital surgeons who demand quick, efficient recovery and discharge and who may rarely visit the facility. The role of nursing home geriatricians shrinks in the face of the surgeons' dictates. Even their continuing responsibility for providing basic background care in the nursing home is squeezed by inadequate reimbursements for their medical direction.

The continuing and even accelerating domination of acute healthcare pervades all levels of housing and services for older people. With the dearth of true geriatric care venues, older adults in the community are left to wend their way through very specialized acute settings. Yet, aging adults, unlike those with only acute conditions,

---

[†] In 2018, only 7,000 of the 985,026 practicing U.S. physicians were geriatricians, and only 50% were practicing full time. The federal model estimates the U.S. will need 33,200 geriatricians by 2025. Therefore, we now have only 10% of the need projected in a few years. And there is little hope for relief in the future. More than one-third of the 384 available slots for graduate fellowships in geriatrics went unfilled in 2019. (Castelucci, M. Geriatrics still failing to attract more doctors. *Modern healthcare*. February 27, 2018. https://www.modernhealthcare.com/article/20180227/NEWS/180229926/geriatrics-still-failing-to-attract-new-doctors)

need permeable borders that allow them to flow through from interventions for chronic issues to treatments for acute problems and back again in order to access the changing resources they need. It is past time that the victory over infectious diseases and the arrival of a new epidemiologic era of multiple chronic conditions in older age is acknowledged and addressed.

As we had learned 30 years earlier when we designed and moved into our New Home, the misery experienced in old, traditional nursing homes was not senescence itself, but in large measure the unintended consequence of outdated delivery systems. Each component of care that we wanted to address and to integrate into a broader kind of care, we found, had been based on an Industrial Age assembly-line model, exemplified by a med cart traveling down a narrow hallway dispensing medications. The medical successes of the 20th century resulted in a dramatic increase of long lives, but no real attention has yet been given to maintaining the quality of life for those who need ongoing orchestration of interventions during those additional years.

Paying for Care

Our society professes to mandate the right to healthcare, and that principle is meant to include care for its older members. Sadly, care is not distributed fairly, and there are internal hurdles and gaps. However, we don't as a matter of policy say that some people can't have healthcare. With limited exceptions, Medicare provides healthcare insurance coverage for everyone older than 65. Under no imaginable circumstance is that going to change. We may change the name, we may collect and distribute funds differently, we may even limit eligibility to those who can't afford private health insurance, but we are not going to stop providing health insurance to people older than 65. The more important question concerns what that healthcare will look like, and the answer should be driven by how we understand and respond to aging, recognizing that older adults need "care" defined more broadly than it is in our current healthcare system.

We will also keep Social Security. It is deeply integrated into the way working-age Americans plan and frame their lives. Any future that supposes the total elimination of the national pension is not realistic. Despite occasional scare stories in the media, the future of both the Social Security pension and our old-age health insurance program (Medicare) are as certain as sunrise tomorrow. They may cover a bit less or we may resort to delaying the age of eligibility, but the essential commitment to older generations the programs represent will endure.

Medicare and Medicaid spending results from the federalization of old-age healthcare during the past half-century. For people 65 and older, healthcare has been an established fact for more than 50 years, with the federal government picking up the basic cost of healthcare, minus some co-payments, through Medicare and sharing with the states through Medicaid the costs of long-term care for the "poor." With the enormous increase in the 65-and-older segment of the population, even if the costs per medical intervention remain unchanged (which they won't), the cost of caring for people 65 and older will increase by more than 50% over the next 10 years.‡

When a frail older adult can no longer perform the activities of daily living necessary to survive, and family members can't provide care, a nursing home has historically been the only answer. The average yearly cost of a private nursing home bed in 2021 was $107,000.[37] Because many residents cannot pay from their own funds, 35% of total federal outlays ($6.6 trillion) in 2020 were for older adults: $765 million for Medicare, $458 million for Medicaid (not including the state share), and $1.1 trillion for Social Security.[38]

Those calculations are for all people over 65. But the really astounding predictions about health expenditures for Medicare and Medicaid are for those over 85. In 1900, there were only 122,000 people over 85 years old living in the United States (0.16% of the U.S. population), as compared to 6.6 million in 2020 (2% of the U.S. population) and projected to be 18 million by 2050 (4.5% of the U.S. population).[39] This is 147 times as many people over 85 as compared to my grandfather's time, a mere two generations ago. This is not just incredible; it is literally incomprehensible. Today, as medicine increasingly protects us from acute illness, late life is usually the time when we need the most healthcare. We often live long enough to

---

‡ Medicare outlays are predicted to increase to $1.92 trillion in 2032, from $868 billion in 2021. (https://www.statista.com/statistics/217612/outlays-for-medicare-and-forecast-in-the-us/).

need long-term care or support. Chronic conditions in the late years of life are now the leading cause of healthcare spending. Our millions of 85-year-olds, many with essentially no assets, need health and supportive care that comes at costs beyond their means. This is an utterly different universe of needs than in 1900.

Beyond the increase in the number of people 65 and older, public resources will be challenged by how many will arrive at 65 with scant resources to sustain them in retirement. The median household net worth of people 55 to 65 in 2016 was $140,000, including real estate, which means that half the population will start retirement with less than that amount, barely enough to pay for a year in a nursing home for one person. Furthermore, it's unlikely they will retain that sum through 2 or 3 decades until they accumulate conditions that require extensive care. Demand for public long-term care benefits (Medicaid) will increase both as the population increases and as that population's need increases.

Traditional pensions no longer exist for most workers, who increasingly have to rely on individual retirement savings plans to supplement their Social Security. With the shift from classic defined-benefit pensions to defined-contribution retirement saving plans, the risk is shifted from the corporate pension fund to the individual. The average monthly Social Security payment in January 2020 was $1,503, or about $18,000 a year.[40] According to Nova (2018), "Nearly one third of Baby Boomers had no money saved in retirement plans in 2014, when they were on average 58 years old."[41] To quote the Stanford Center on Longevity, "compared to older generations, Baby Boomers have accrued less savings and more debt, putting them in an especially vulnerable position as they move through retirement."[42] What does that mean for that average retiree whose spouse needs care that costs $100,000 a year? Three-quarters of the population of Baby Boomers will not be well financed in retirement or able to buy into retirement communities, assisted living facilities, or long-term care. A large population will retire with no assets at all. The money, private or public, to pay their bills doesn't seem to be there.

A 2022 study reveals that "more than 100 million people in America, including 41% of adults (are) beset by a health system that is systematically pushing patients into debt on a mass scale."[43] The nation's collective medical debt is an estimated \$200 billion.[44] The highest medical debt is in areas with high rates of multiple chronic diseases. The amounts owed are often hidden from view because they are included in "credit card balances, loans from family, or payment plans to hospitals and other medical providers."[45] The scale of unmet financial obligations comes to dominate older peoples' lives.

Neither the government nor individuals currently have the resources to deal with the costs of care for an older population of the size that exists today and is still growing. Projecting the current trends forward, we are out of money and labor and heading for a crash of some kind in Medicare and Medicaid. We are facing growing shortfalls of geriatric doctors, nurses, and nursing home beds. Institutions and professions simply cannot evolve rapidly enough to handle the onrush of demand. Even under perfect conditions with joint purpose and cooperation, it would probably take at least 10 years for medical and nursing schools to produce a new cadre of geriatricians and geriatric nurses who understand chronic care. And who knows how long it would take Congress to overhaul legislation dealing with the needs of older adults?

The projections for the time when all the Baby Boomers will have reached age 65 can't be met without very large increases in government revenue. No matter how the projections are set up, even if people live healthier lives and medical costs increase more slowly, the trend lines always end in the zone of unaffordability. That is the crux of the debate about what the nation should do in the future to cover the care needs of the old. Will we collectively assume the costs of aging? Or will we reduce the government resources available to people over 65? So far, our efforts have not touched the real problem because the problem moved while no one was looking. It became the problem of chronic conditions, not the problem of getting older.

Most reforms we have been trying to make to existing programs will be ineffective against the coming financial crunch created by expanding numbers and longevity of older adults. To try to manage the cost of the aging population by reforming medical care is to start from the wrong place. Reform needs to begin with prevention and maintenance rather than with acute care. Prevention and maintenance, particularly of chronic conditions, are among the "cattle" we forgot when we set out on the trail to take care of our oldest members.

The current misguided approach is evident in some of the changes being implemented to try to address the issue of costs. Alterations to reimbursement rules for institutional care, for example, have forced nursing homes to take in more and more frail older clients, who are less able to appreciate their physical environment. This has caused nursing homes to become more medicalized and thus, paradoxically, even more dependent on diminishing governmental funds. As time has passed and the profile of the residents has changed, the kinds of public spaces we carefully calibrated in the New Home have become an extra expense, no longer useful to short-term residents with more acute challenges. External conditions have simply overwhelmed the evolution that had been improving nursing homes for a decade and a half.

To summarize the situation: We know how many very older adults are alive today. We know a lot about how to keep them safe. We also know there will be many more 85- and 90-year-olds in the population 10 years from now. We can estimate their needs. A growing number of frail older people are likely to have multiple chronic conditions, less physical and mental vigor, and increasing dependence on environmental supports. But many of the systems we use to deliver medical care to this new population are archaic. They were built to treat acute diseases in a younger, more resilient population and are not suited to head off and address flare-ups of chronic conditions in an older, frail population.

Until we can see what's around us in the world of chronic conditions correlated with aging, we can't address the issues that dominate that world. Whether we respond appropriately depends on whether we face this changed relationship with health. Until we do, given the mismatch between our behaviors and the new reality, we will suffer discomfort and face financial overruns.

We discovered with the New Home 30 years ago that the familiar sights, sounds, and smells were not the result of inherent senescence, but instead were the consequence of inappropriate delivery systems. We need to repeat this lesson for the new cohort of frail older adults. Tens of millions of Boomers are entering into uncharted decades of their lives and into uncharted territory without an accurate map or the tools to fashion their journey. They will be the ones to demand and create a new world of aging.

Conclusion

We have defined the fundamental problem. We are living through a transition in the demographics and life experience that began a decade or so ago, with a rapidly expanding older population, most of them with chronic conditions. It will probably take another 2 decades before we have fully absorbed the change. Our healthcare system can't take care of the new older cohort properly and couldn't afford to even if it were set up to do so. In fact, the health system that is supposed to be a support may actually act as a drain that sucks the possibilities out of life in older age. In the following chapters, I will describe how I believe that problem is going to be addressed.

CHAPTER 10

Solving the Problem

The Law of Interchangeable Interventions

The description of Mrs. Smith in the Introduction is an illustration of how a solution to caring for older adults will be constructed for one individual. By expanding the use of technology exponentially, as was done for her, we will create a new world of aging. This evolution will come about because of a number of forces, the most important of which is a phenomenon that I call the Law of Interchangeable Interventions. Its role is so central to the future of aging in the United States that this chapter is devoted to it.

Traditionally, we have placed frail older people who need help and who aren't in the care of family into institutions. As we have seen, nursing homes were, and mostly still are, factories of care, operating on an industrial model of batch processing and economies of scale, rather than on individualized needs and preferences. This system is no longer viable, however, not only because coming generations will not accept its dehumanizing conditions, but also because the number of older men and women and the length of their lives have made institutional care prohibitively expensive.

Some changes in the care of older adults can already be seen in small ways. Perhaps your 92-year-old mother hasn't had a fall, and she hasn't yet been in a hospital. In fact, other than arthritis, poor eyesight, and needing to steady herself with a walker, she's pretty healthy. She makes her own breakfast, but she gets a Meals on Wheels delivery that you easily arrange for her online. She follows an exercise video on YouTube that she learned about in her doctor's office. She visits with you or one of your siblings on some kind of video chat almost every day. Ten years ago, she would probably have needed to be in a licensed residential care setting, at much greater expense, in order to get food and exercise. She would have talked to distant family members only occasionally. Thirty years ago, she would have been even more isolated in a nursing home. Today, older adults are searching out countless options that create a way of life that won't break the bank or the spirit.

The Law of Interchangeable Interventions

Given a choice between care in a family setting and care in a nursing home, most people choose family. Given a choice between living with their adult children or staying in their own home, most older people prefer to maintain control and independence and do not wish to be a burden, which leads them to choose remaining in their own home.[46] As we will see in more detail as we proceed, interventions in the environment can now provide the assistance needed for older people to live safely at home for much longer than has ever been possible. This trend is continuing as the number of available interventions increases. Various options can be substituted for one another according to the person's needs and preferences to produce approximately the same outcome. When this happens, the options can be considered interchangeable.

From 40 years of working with people who need help with their living arrangements and their health as their bodies age, I have come to realize a certain basic pattern. When we face a need for assistance and have a range of choices, human behavior is consistent. From the available and effective interventions, the *least expensive, least medicalized, and most consistent with a person's pre-senescent life* is the most desirable. I call this drive to find the option that is economical and palatable, while remaining satisfyingly effective, the Law of Interchangeable Interventions.

Interventions that change a condition and improve an outcome are not confined to medicine. Putting grab bars in the bathroom is an intervention, as is a telephone that connects to hearing aids. Interventions that fill in for changes associated with age, furthermore, don't exist in isolation from one another. The more accommodating the environment, the less assistance it takes to get around in it. When frailty enters, if we intervene to overcome the effects of disability, we can maintain a living situation for a longer period of time. When we do need help, if we've equipped ourselves well and had the resources to build our environment right, we need less assistance than we would have otherwise. The Law of Interchangeable Interventions urges us to choose the methods that will make a difference in the least expensive and least disruptive ways. And when it becomes necessary to make further changes, we will compromise where we must, but we prefer to concede as little as possible. That is how people behave when given the option to do so. Unfortunately, this has often not been the path offered by many healthcare providers, who may not be aware of available interventions outside of their own areas of specialization.

The Law of Interchangeable Interventions suggests, for example, that frail older adults can receive many of the interventions they need in a variety of settings, not just nursing in homes. It encourages us to choose, if at all possible without putting people at unnecessary risk, less confining environments rather than more restrictive ones, less costly solutions rather than more expensive ones, and less invasive procedures rather than more medicalized ones. Some frail residents can be moved out of nursing homes into specialized housing that is less expensive to build and operate. Many design and technology innovations developed in nursing homes are already being inserted into housing for older residents or integrated into people's homes, enabling us to support some frail people safely in more independent settings. A device that can send an emergency message to a caregiver, for example, is the digital version of a nurse call cord that is only available to the client in a nursing home if he or she stays near the bed.

In addition to technologies that allow frail adults to stay longer in their own homes, safe and appropriate placements for those who can no longer live on their own will increase in number and compete in the marketplace. The choices they offer will respond to ever more fine gradations in clients' competencies, supported by new interventions. In housing stock that was inflexible, for example, there was great risk that a particular loss, such as needing a wheelchair, could push a person out of an independent-living arrangement into a more medicalized environment. This segregated the frail older adults, placing them together in homogeneous settings with little attention to individual preferences. Now they have the option, because other living arrangements have become safer, of choosing to remain in a less expensive and less medicalized environment, and they happily do so. The result of greater flexibility in housing is greater diversity and enrichment for older people and the community.

In addition to design innovations, there are many other categories of interventions available to members of the older populations. Exercise and diet can be miracle drugs. Specialized routines can profoundly affect the course of a person's aging. A new lifestyle and wellness industry is beginning to compete with the traditional crisis-oriented health system, ameliorating some of the chronic conditions that afflict many older adults and reducing acute incidents.

Imagine a person who becomes persistently sad and listless and goes to the doctor for help. The doctor diagnoses the problem as depression. He or she could offer a list of interventions that have been proven effective, sorted by cost and medical intrusiveness, ranging from taking a brisk walk to sitting in front of a special light box, more social engagement, counseling, medication, a hospital stay, and even electric shock therapy. These options aren't entirely interchangeable, of course, because a less medically oriented intervention such as exercise will not work for someone in a deep clinical depression. They are partially interchangeable, however, in the sense that all of them are possible options to reduce depression. Too often, however, the person is offered only the interventions at the end of the list, the more expensive and medically oriented ones, since they are the ones with which the doctor is most familiar and because choosing them is incentivized by existing payment systems.

The Law of Interchangeable Interventions should, and often does, also shape the approach of the payer. Ideally, taxpayers, insurance premium payers, and the government will prefer the least expensive among an array of comparably effective interventions. Because medical interventions are frequently more expensive than their social equivalents, the desire of families and third-party payers will often align. Both will want to find the option that is effective while also being, as described previously, the least expensive, least medicalized, and most consistent with pre-senescent life. It is this confluence of interests that makes the Law of Interchangeable Interventions the dominant dynamic in the aging world.

We don't usually think of frail adults as active consumers. But as they become aware of more consumer choices, competition for their business is creating a huge new market. We're already spending more than a trillion dollars a year on interventions of all sorts. Much of what happens in that market is already affected by the Law of Interchangeable Interventions, so that the provider who produces a less expensive, less medicalized intervention to meet a particular need will get more business.

Inside, Outside, Beside

To see in more detail how aging will work when the Law of Interchangeable Interventions is utilized to fuller effect, it may be useful to consider interventions in three categories: interventions that work *Inside* the body, such as food and medications; ones that provide help from *Outside* of the body, such as braces and wheelchairs; and ones that exist *Beside* the older adult, like a granddaughter or an aide, who can steady him or her with a hand on the elbow or an encouraging word.

Inside Interventions

In my lifetime, we have seen a radical proliferation of innovative Inside interventions. Imaging, for example, has evolved from x-rays in the 1950s to CAT scans and laser cameras today. We can see inside the body in incredible detail and detect problems earlier, when they may be more readily resolved. We also benefit from new drug designs based on discoveries in molecular biology and genetics. From 1970 to 2021, life expectancy in the United States improved by 5.32 years,[47] in some measure because of medical innovations.[48] Some of these medications don't remove the problem entirely, but they maintain and improve function. New medications for arthritis, for example, interfere with the progression of the illness so that we can hold the condition at bay. In more and more circumstances, if I take a particular pill I can continue to live in my apartment, satisfying one of the principles of the Law of Interchangeable Interventions: the desire to maintain a life as consistent as possible with the life I have had.

In addition to chemical and imaging interventions, there are artificial body parts, organ transplants, and cataract operations. We can tune up our vision with laser surgery or insert a pacemaker to keep the heart on a regular beat. Hip replacements have become routine, numbering 400,000 in the United States in 2018, and recovery from the surgery is rapid. It is projected that by 2030 hip replacements will increase 71% and knee replacements 84.9%.[49] Before these surgeries were available, lameness from arthritic hips and damaged knees might distort the entire body as it twisted to cope with a painful joint. If we stop walking because of pain or lack of balance, the consequences are serious. Digestion slows down, muscles begin to atrophy, and inactivity leads to loss of appetite and even depression. Now, with the option of joint replacement, the person once condemned to a painful slide toward immobility can look forward to climbing stairs, walking, and even biking, recovering the life he or she knew before. The person is also walking away, at least for some years, from a need for protracted periods of expensive long-term care.

From the outside, no one can tell who is a "bionic" man or woman and who isn't. The fusion of humans and machines that can be found today in research labs, hospitals, and streets in the United States are producing what are referred to as "Techno Sapiens." [50] Researchers are exploring ways to repair, refurbish, or replace human organs, from 3D printing to growing an artificial heart.[51] Pulitzer Prize-winning sociobiologist Edward O. Wilson stated, "We're about to abandon natural selection, the process that created us, in order to direct our own evolution by volitional selection—the process of redirecting our biology and human nature as we wish them to be."[52] These dramatic and often newly available Inside innovations improve how older people function and mitigate the accumulation of interacting losses that lead to decline, expensive institutional care, and death.

Outside Interventions

A second category of innovations resides in the environment around and outside of us, which is being rethought and reshaped to support older adults' needs. Fixtures, furniture, carpets and lighting can be adapted to make up for many. Television remotes were originally designed for anyone who would rather not get off the couch, but they are also a boon for someone who is unable to stand up. Remotes controlled by voice command can be connected to switches for lamps and power window shades, as well as an Internet connection and a cell phone, allowing an older adult who has trouble moving around to accomplish a number of tasks on his or her own, almost as easily as when he or she was physically capable. He or she no longer needs the staff of a nursing home to get through the day.

In 1990, Sam Farber noticed that his wife, who had mild arthritis, was having difficulty gripping ordinary kitchen tools. He and his son designed 15 different gadgets that were easier to hold and use. They introduced them at the Gourmet Products Show in San Francisco under the name of OXO Good Grips. In 2004, the company was valued at $273 million. Today, OXO offers more than 1,000 products, all of them tools that are easier and more comfortable for everybody to use.[53] In particular, they allow older cooks to manage their kitchen tasks by themselves for many additional years. The market jumped at these new interventions, which are much less expensive than hiring a cook, and allowed an important aspect of the customer's life to continue without disruption. The Law of Interchangeable Interventions, seeking better alternatives, drove the inventions and their success.

Replacing doorknobs with levers is another simple change that eliminates a barrier imposed by reduced motor functioning in older age. A lever is easier to work than a knob because it doesn't have to be grasped with arthritic fingers. In the past, being unable to open the door might have been seen as one more bit of evidence that a parent couldn't live alone any longer. With a technology available at every store that sells doorknobs and a bit of marketing to the older consumer, the problem is no longer a threat to independence. Installing new door hardware is a lot less expensive than moving to an assisted living facility. The same is true for higher toilet seats, modified shower compartments, wide doorways, stair gliders, and powered scooters. The world is a cornucopia of interventions, many of which were available long before their advantages for older adults were recognized.

Any nursing home serves as a showroom of Outside interventions that can be extended to work in a private home. Modern nursing home carpeting, for example, is engineered to fulfill multiple specialized needs. It reduces the likelihood of falls and lessens the damage from falls that do occur. It lets wheelchairs and walkers roll easily and is backed with material impervious to spills that can be especially problematic when incontinence is an issue. It's even easy to clean. It was developed and sold by the healthcare divisions of carpet manufacturers, but when the companies see the consumer market for the product, we can be sure that we'll find it in the home division in any color anyone might want. Many products developed for institutions are finding everyday applications for individual consumers in large numbers, just as items developed for the space program have become available to the general public. The Law of Interchangeable Interventions determines the success of each innovation.

A wheelchair with a smaller radius can reduce the size needed for the bathroom. Bathrooms for adults with mobility issues used to be cavernous, designed for cumbersome wheelchairs with a large turning radius. Today, wheelchairs can practically turn on their own axes and can navigate into tiny spaces without bumping into fixtures or walls. A small bathroom in the home a person has lived in for a long time becomes usable and is comfortingly familiar for private moments. Relocation to a specialized facility is not necessary.

All the functions of daily life are currently subjects of intense investigation toward finding ways to stretch an older adult's competencies. In essence, we are asking the environment to reach out to meet and complement people's capacities, with less expense and disruption. As the demand for such devices grows, more and more products, from Velcro shoe fasteners to talking microwave ovens, will come onto the market or extend their usefulness to the oldest generation.

Beside Interventions

A third large category of interventions in caring for older people is made up of the human supports that combine with Inside processes and Outside mechanical support systems. The helping hand at the bedside is a kind of assistance that's as old as humankind. Although there is nothing like the touch of another human being, it is expensive. Direct caregiving requires the presence of the caregiver along with his or her physical and mental exertion. The monetary value of the help families provide, usually for free, to aging parents or spouses was estimated to be $522 billion a year in 2014.[54] This is 2.5 times more than the amount spent on formal long-term care, including nursing homes, home health aides, and adult day services. In recent years, however, this historic economic resource has become insufficient to deal with the much larger number of frail older adults in the community. More women have entered the workforce or have moved away and are no longer available to care for older relatives. Families are smaller and cannot spread the responsibilities as widely among their members, as seen in the demographics discussed in Chapter 1. This coincides, unfortunately, with a multiplying number who need care as well as an increase in their years of needing it because they are living longer.

Traditional human Beside services must become more efficient as we strive to reduce the costs of aging. Greater use of Inside and Outside interventions will help. For example, camera monitoring can dramatically reduce the time needed for the physical proximity of caregivers. In fact, the helping hand at the bedside is the intervention that will experience the most visible change as the future of aging unfolds. If I correct my poor vision, replace the old gas stove with a simple microwave, and set myself up to get my groceries delivered, then I don't need someone to come in and cook for me, and I may not even need Meals on Wheels. If my health status is sent automatically over the Internet every day so that my weight, blood pressure, glucose levels, and even urine are automatically checked for problematic changes, an aide doesn't need to visit to collect the information. The digital report eliminates the costs of the driver who takes me to the health clinic, the staff who checks me in, and the nurse who makes the reading. The hands-on contact of a health worker will be provided when something looks wrong, but not for many of the services they perform now. Therefore, I consume less labor, get a less invasive intervention, and save some money. More of my visitors will be the loved ones I really want to see, and they will not have to spend their time on caregiving chores instead of enjoying my company.

Compounding Inside, Outside, and Beside Interventions

Digital networks equipped with sensors, screens, and audio will reduce the need to concentrate older adults in one place unless they are bed bound or have severe dementia or other mental illness. Some rural areas may not have adequate access to networks right away, but for much of the United States, monitoring can be remote and automatic. Attendants will not need to be present except when necessary. In the Industrial Age, assembly-line economies of scale made it less expensive to build nursing homes that delivered factory-style care than to provide individual care settings for every person who needed assistance. Digital technology has reversed that. The economies of scale and efficiencies of the assembly-line system have been overwhelmed by diseconomies of scale, building costs, and the burdensome, repetitive tasks imposed on the institutional staff.

This shift is my most important message to the reader. With all the environmental interventions that support the capabilities of people, staying at home is becoming ever more frequently the much less expensive alternative, as well as the most desirable. New interventions, whether Inside, Outside, or Beside, are continuously remodeling the environment for older people. An innovation in any of the three categories can have direct ripple effects on the other two. If an Outside innovation has real impact, it should change both the way the individual functions (Inside), as well as reduce or change his or her service needs (Beside). The lighter wheelchair with a smaller turning radius (Outside) not only reduces the square footage necessary in a bathroom, but it can relieve a homecare aide of transferring the person to the toilet (Beside) because the person can now get close enough to transfer him- or herself. It also allows the person in the wheelchair to extend his or her repertories of tasks, resulting in increased exercise and emotional self-worth (Inside). As the wheelchair becomes less obtrusive, the person presents more normalized responses to the world and engages more fully in social interactions, which has enormous emotional and psychological benefits.

Some interventions fall into more than one category. The Internet is an Inside intervention when it is used for telemedicine, such as logging vital signs into a database for daily automatic review, and a Beside intervention that sets up a video appointment with a nurse, a social worker, or an accountant.

When interventions are successful, such as when you are so comfortable with the backup camera in your car that you are no longer aware it replaced craning your neck and allowed you to continue to drive, that intervention becomes an unconscious extension of yourself into the external world. It's no wonder that this cascade of interventions, coming from almost every angle, competing and setting up new opportunities for ever-newer interventions, is too ubiquitous to be visible.

Interventions generally get our attention only when our limitations or those of someone we're caring for demand we find one. The

Law of Interchangeable Interventions plays out so effectively in the lives of older adults that we don't always realize how actively they are involved in shaping their own destinies by choosing among interventions. The increasing presence of more active and competent older people indicates how the Law of Interchangeable Interventions is functioning.

Conclusion

The fact that many frail older adults are making consumer choices, and that the market is responding to them, has transferred a portion of their care back into their own hands. As we develop more interventions, we are slowly coming to realize that many of the conditions we assumed were an unavoidable part of aging can actually be mitigated. The locus of control in aging has moved from controlled environments like nursing homes to places and services that cater to the individual's wishes and respond to his or her control, and to the person him- or herself.

PART III

Our Future Aging Experience

CHAPTER 11

We're Not Bankrupt

*The Future of Aging Through the Lens of the
Law of Interchangeable Interventions*

I have been concerned with the present and the past in the last several chapters in order to demonstrate why we don't see aging as it is now, why we didn't see the enormous demographic growth of older adults, and why we deal with the needs of the frail aging population the way we do today. I hope that seeing aging as it actually is today and knowing its history is useful in considering how the situation will evolve. Each of us will deal with aging on a personal level, through parents, spouses, friends, or ourselves, and aging is also one of the most important issues for the nation to confront now and in the future.

The book opened with a view of how things might be in the near future if we finally come to understand today's aging and begin to deal with it more realistically. Our existing worldview based on the ways things were in the past doesn't help us understand its interlocking phenomena. We need to develop a dynamic concept of the world of aging that creates a web of relationships between ideas, people, and processes. I also pinpointed the most serious problem standing in our way as our insufficient attention to the chronic conditions that have come to dominate older adults' health. Twentieth-century acute care medicine, with its big hospitals and emphasis on curing diseases and saving lives, is being overtaken by the needs and extent of chronic conditions that require attention. In 2020, "The Centers for Disease Control and Prevention (CDC) estimated that 90% of national healthcare spending goes toward chronic condition management and mental health care."[55] As acute care inevitably makes way for chronic care, a whole new toolbox of interventions, ranging from streaming exercise programs to talking pill bottles, is entering the stage. All these interventions compete for the business of older consumers, who make choices based on the fundamental principle of the Law of Interchangeable Interventions, as described in Chapter 10: to go on living as closely as possible to the life they have been living at the lowest possible cost. With so many new interventions available, many older people will be able to stay at home.

The new world of interventions can transform care for an aging populace far beyond what most people realize. Many innovations now allow care to be provided by less highly trained and less expensive caregivers. A nurse or aide or even the client him- or herself can sometimes do what used to be the purview of the doctor. If a highly trained medical professional is not necessary at all times, care can then move out of traditional health settings. As new innovations allow someone to obtain care at home, sleeping accommodations can become disconnected from medical and programmatic needs, and substantial portions of care can relocate. More older adults can remain in their own communities. The number of residential facilities is already shrinking. "Nationally, 200 to 300 nursing homes close each year," according to Nicholas Castle, as reported to Paula Span. Span continued, "the number of residents keeps shrinking, too, from 1.48 million in 2000 to 1.36 million in 2015, according to federal data."[56]

From the perspective of the old paradigm, if we continue to pay today's healthcare expenses, we will soon be bankrupt, facing impossible shortfalls as the aging cohort grows. But the truth is that we're not bankrupt. The United States is flush with resources to solve this problem. They're just not where we've been accustomed to looking for them. As should be clear from the many examples that have already been cited, interventions no longer need to come only from the traditional healthcare centers. The food, energy, labor, and transportation already in our communities can also be adapted to integrate frail adults. My woeful description in Chapter 3 of the potential calamity caused by demographics, strained resources, and our inflexible management of aging care delivery has one major fault. It assumes that the way we deliver aging care won't change. In reality, the old way can and will be transformed by digital technology. Rather than assuming that a demographic wave will engulf the nation and consume most of its resources, I believe it is actually more likely that the Law of Interchangeable Interventions will produce a manageable future.

This future is already coming into sight. Both cost, which is a key element in the Law of Interchangeable Interventions, and knowledge, which expands consumer choice, are pulling healthcare and aging care onto the web. This migration should move the power to choose interventions and to demand competitive costs, now closely held in the citadels of medicine, into the hands of older people and their families.

Older adults already have an increasing number of options that they can assemble into new outcomes for themselves, according to the Law of Interchangeable Interventions. The transition to less expensive and less invasive care will not be neat, coordinated, or predictable. We can already see interventions leapfrog one another and appear from unexpected directions, impacting present practice in surprising ways. In this exciting landscape, older people and their families will hunt for bargains among the interventions that can change their lives.

Remember that the market for supplies and services for people in their later years is becoming large enough to have an impact on the nation's economy, as it races to accommodate demands for clothing, carpets, lights, furniture, electronics, and other products attractive to aging consumers. Buildings are ceasing to be the largest expense in providing care for older adults, giving way to the development and management of care options and networks that coordinate technological, physical, and human resources. We need to stop expecting the trajectory of the aging experience to look like it used to so that we can see what is actually happening.

Although we will not retreat from the principle of universal healthcare for people over 65, there is no social commitment to providing care in institutions, especially if less expensive alternatives are available. People who can pay for nursing home care generally don't want it if there's any alternative. A new world of aging is self-assembling even now from components that didn't exist a few years ago, combined with techniques we have known forever. As care devolves from complicated, expensive institutional settings, such as hospitals and nursing homes, to less rigorously formal interventions, such as ambulatory health centers and home healthcare, costs will go down.

A Digital Database

A major factor in the creation of many of the new innovations available is digital technology. We can now collect, communicate, and process data efficiently. Network communication offers continuous, real-time monitoring and reporting, effectively eliminating the need to collect clients in one place. We can monitor vital signs and talk with anyone from any location. We can check how often the refrigerator has been opened or whether pills have been dispensed. All this information can flow through a database that continuously updates a person's health or physical status. The same technology allows light fixtures, window shades, thermostats, and home security to be operated remotely or automatically. If a person can no longer get up to open the front door to admit a caregiver, he or she can unlock the door remotely.

Consider, as another example, what might happen to the medical chart. A generation ago, a physician heard a patient's complaints, made notes in his or her chart, and then announced the next steps. On the next office visit, the doctor picked up the chart and continued the notes where he or she had left off. The chart was a record of the client's status; the client never saw the chart. It was filed in a chart room with a few thousand others. The doctor owned it. Now, an alternative exists in the form of a digital chart. Continually updated health information can be displayed in any format. The patient can see test results at home. The doctor's office can send relevant notes to the pharmacy or to technicians doing tests. All medical interactions and results are automatically added.

Although the physician is already using an electronic health record, we can carry the concept further to improve the lives of older adults. The present chart is an improvement on the paper file of the past, but it is available only to a fairly limited group of participants. When physicians want to connect to other doctors or to hospitals and labs, they still have to solve problems involving security, privacy, and the incompatibility of different systems. And they have no connections to other services that a client receives, such as food deliveries or massage therapy.

We already have the technology to create a much more comprehensive network. Medicare has figured out how to collect and process information on 45 million members, including all the office visits, tests, procedures, prescriptions, hospitalizations, physical therapy, gym memberships, and more, for the purpose of reimbursing providers. To help the healthcare system evaluate appropriate care plans, a comprehensive chart that gathers information from many sources could be programmed to compare one person's medical details anonymously with everyone else's and then provide a wide range of useful information on the successes and failures of interventions used for cases with the same features. The super database I am advocating will have embedded in it, anonymously, the experiences of millions of patients, the entirety of medical literature, and the interventions selected by tens of thousands of physicians. It can look at the roads others have traveled and report on the results of various treatments and interventions, helping caregivers to make decisions for individuals.

The database can expand beyond the traditional limits of medical information to include any information that might be useful in maintaining an older adult's well-being. Imagine this super chart loaded with all the places in one's community that serve hot lunches, sortable by distance or menu options; all the means of local transportation available, sortable by price or type of vehicle or schedule; and all personal assistance programs available in a community from ATMs to beauty salons.

Digital data analysis now makes it possible to find useful information within previously daunting quantities of data. Information generated by older adults using transportation, food delivery, or in-home blood pressure devices will fill up databases of consumer behavior like the ones online retailers use. Digitized data analysis will reveal which among comparable interventions is less costly but as effective as others. It will be possible, for example, to determine if a home visit from a housekeeper trained to care for someone with moderate dementia is more or less disorienting to a particular person than a visit to an adult day center would be. Network communication in the form of social media can put small communities of family members or neighbors in continuous contact so designated people are aware if anyone is sick or struggling. These social media components reduce the need to be face-to-face to find out if help is needed.

Looking at all the information we collect and collate about health and aging will reveal new or better ways to stay healthy. It's also probable that, with enough data, we'll see where costs in healthcare are out of line with their effects. If, for example, there is enough data to prove definitely that two drugs produce the same results and the same side effects, but one drug is significantly more expensive, then choosing the less expensive drug will be easy and uncontroversial. Data may reveal the same kind of opportunity for saving with social interventions. Perhaps it will turn out that homecare is a healthier option for a certain set of frail older adults than social day care, or the other way around.

It is still the case today that when the doctor reviews a set of symptoms, he or she will probably recommend a course based on his or her experience and judgment. That usually works pretty well. An aggregation of millions of such cases with the results of various treatments for the doctor to consider before making a recommendation could work even better.

Here is my rosy projection of the future: In the face of accumulating chronic conditions in the aging population, the primary question for both consumers and insurers of healthcare and aging care will be, just as it is now, how to find the right balance of interventions and cost. With a database that includes the entire population of Medicare-covered persons, answers to that question will be increasingly refined, with the result that we will live longer and less expensively. The intellectual and emotional power of the doctor's office and the hospital as unique seats of medical wisdom will be diminished by the loss of their exclusivity. The aggregation of more and more information about everyone, collected from medical records, from sensors at home in smart houses, and in our ubiquitous handheld devices, will make effective preventive protocols stand out. Signs of incipient conditions will stand out more brightly and lead to earlier interventions.

This might sound fanciful, but the technologies I'm assuming in my picture of the digital future of healthcare and aging care all exist today, just as the technologies that produced the smartphone were either available or foreseeable in the 20 years before anyone except science fiction writers imagined them. The network-enabled future makes the environment intelligent and supportive, which reduces the emotional impact of physical and cognitive losses associated with aging by slowing them down and making them easier to live with, and that makes aging less difficult and less noticeable. You can continue to be in a State of Benescence, and you can continue in it longer.

The more interventions that are introduced, the more competition there will be among them. The more competition among interventions, the more surely the more effective, less costly, less medical, less compromising interventions will emerge from among the alternatives. That's the ideal.

So, what might be negatives to this rosy future? Privacy will be a major concern, as already noted. The different health and care systems for the aging populations of the 50 different states will bring their own local interests and twists, but I'm convinced that we will find our way with these new tools. We will learn to use them with increasing refinement; we'll solve the problems slowly but surely. The Industrial Age is already over, even though we don't always realize it. Digital technology is supplanting it, and it's time we started taking advantage of that in aging and healthcare, as we have in so many other dimensions of our lives.

Privacy Considerations

When older adults read the description in this book of a future networked home, with devices collecting many bits of private information, caregivers tracking visits on their cell phones, and communication between providers and family members, many will cry, "I won't give up my privacy! Too many people will see too much about me! I'd rather be left alone!" While this is understandable, an older person should stop and consider a few things before turning away.

Much of the information that will be shared in the networked environment is already in the computer systems of an older adult's healthcare providers. There, it is protected from inappropriate prying eyes by HIPAA regulations. The same protections will apply to systems installed in a person's home. Information will be accessible only to those who have been designated by the client.

Furthermore, it is often older adults' desire for privacy that becomes a threat to the independence they want to achieve. It cuts them off from accessing the treasure trove of interventions that could enable them to retain a greater degree of function and true independence. In the present system, the data reside elsewhere: at the doctor's office, the hospital, the pharmacy. The usefulness of this information is limited, and it belongs to someone else. An unfortunate consequence of refusing to share data may be the very consequence that is most feared, institutionalization. When a person is forced to leave his or her home for a congregated setting, the insult to privacy is much more severe. Few older men and women wish to trade their homes for a shared room, to eat meals in groups, and live within routines dictated by others. Traditionally, such congregated settings have been the only environments where a full panoply of services for frail residents was available. In those settings, even one's shared bedroom is constantly penetrated by caregivers in order for them to gather information and deliver services. This may be experienced as a loss of dignity and of one's (former) identity.

In contrast, digitization, even though it involves sharing some information, will enable a person to keep personal control over how the information is used. Investing the private home with small-scale Inside, Outside, and Beside interventions that remove many of the risks previously left unattended will reduce the threat of placement in a nursing home. The data can be fed privately and seamlessly to algorithms that analyze and suggest tailored changes only to individuals the person selects. Then, the administration of selected interventions can be facilitated.

Such supportive network systems are already around us in other dimensions of our lives. While grocery stores, banks, transportation, entertainment, and shopping may seem unchanged, they are actually tied to networked systems that invisibly track our individual purchases and activities and make suggestions about goods and services based on our behavior.

Conclusion

Networks can reveal and transform many of the changes now routinely correlated with age to conditions that can be addressed. The ongoing feedback can occur seamlessly and unobtrusively. The digitized environment will enable people to remain safely at home, where they wish to live. The cost of independence is sharing information and taking individual responsibility for the opportunities that are available, but the reward is a lifestyle that reflects one's individual preferences.

CHAPTER 12

Business Enters the Stage

Primarily because of digital technology, life for older adults is already sufficiently changed to suggest that a new age has already begun for them. The digital tools we now possess can help with their daily life and capabilities. The job at hand is to assure that technology continues to change the nature of how and where aging care services are delivered, so that we end up with a system that is both more satisfactory and affordable. The interventions older clients use and the organizations they interact with need to come together ever more strongly to free them more and more from the physical limitations of the pre-digital world and relieve increasing numbers of older people from being presented with a stark choice between independence and institutionalization.

In sectors of the economy outside of aging, the world has already witnessed such revolutions. In retailing, for example, online shopping has disrupted the old model that was based on physical stores. An online store can offer better prices, a bigger selection, and fast delivery. Amazon started as an online retailer of books and wiped out many bookstores, which shook up the book-publishing industry and then, in fairly short order, almost all retailing. Digital technology and retail sales converged to produce something new: retail without physical locations. This convergence in turn transformed other businesses, such as package-delivery services. The elimination of physical limitations gave a company such as Amazon the opportunity to expand beyond the book business into other retail products, even food. Other companies can offer competitive choices. The consumer finds what is needed from a wide array of available options. There is no longer any loyalty to, or even awareness of, traditional suppliers in historic industrial sectors or delivery systems.

Tech Companies and Healthcare

Healthcare, the sector of the economy that consumes almost 18% of our gross domestic product, has not taken full advantage of this kind of innovation and competition, especially those vendors of healthcare that come from outside its historic sector boundaries, primarily because of the historic laws and regulations that govern every aspect of it. But healthcare is finally beginning to attract business innovators who would like a piece of its multi-trillion-dollar market. Care for older adults, including custodial care, is certainly a plum worth reaching to pluck. As Scott Galloway, professor at New York University's Stern School of Business, explained to James D. Walsh, big tech companies have no choice but to enter the healthcare arena. In order to retain their stockholders, big tech needs to increase its revenues substantially, but there are few arenas where that increase is possible. Galloway said,

> Big tech companies . . . have to go big game hunting. You can't feed a city raising squirrels. Those big tech companies have to turn their eyes to new prey, the list of which gets pretty short pretty fast if you look at how big these industries need to be in that weight class . . . government, education and health.[57]

In fact, in a series of multi-billion-dollar acquisitions, mergers, and joint ventures, major players from different traditional sectors, each with its own developmental pathway, seem to be starting to approach aging in the Digital Age by connecting currently separate segments that address different parts of the issue. As of this writing, several retail companies (e.g., Walgreens, Walmart, CVS, and Amazon) have partnered with healthcare insurers (e.g., UnitedHealth and Aetna), technology companies (e.g., Microsoft, Care Centrix, Optum, and CareMark Rx), and care providers (e.g.,VillageMD, Signify, and One Medical) to enhance the range of services they can provide.[58-61]

These mergers and alliances will combine the cultures of distinctly different organizations and can be seen as the beginning of a lead up to the major challenge of caring for older adults. Virtually all of the resources being combined, however, were designed for acute care in the Industrial Age and will require conversion if they are to embark upon the kind of multidisciplinary engagement with chronic care that this book envisions. Traditional specialization and economies of scale must be inverted to align with the Law of Interchangeable Interventions, and a whole new universe of actors must be created. New corporate frameworks, finances, algorithms, and care providers will be precursors to the reorientation of American society to a new relationship with its oldest citizens.

Business innovators interested in the healthcare market, including the sector aimed at the older population, will undoubtedly begin to take advantage of the Law of Interchangeable Interventions. They will recognize opportunities to earn a share of the healthcare sector by introducing interchangeable interventions to attract customers. Companies might enter anew the business of being healthcare providers.

Here's how big tech companies might change the picture of how we pay for healthcare. Imagine two groups, of whatever size is considered large enough to provide reliable information, each including randomly selected 65- to 95-year-olds from the same community. Address the healthcare costs of one group using the traditional Industrial Age model of healthcare delivery with payments coming from existing private or governmental insurers. This is the control group. For the other, experimental group, provide extensive intervention options, as if they were enrolled in a gigantic PACE program (the program described in Chapter 7 that provides all health and long-term care services for a fixed fee per enrollee) with the objective of minimizing hospitalizations and nursing home stays, and of finding the least expensive and invasive options.

In this experiment, we utilize a very large digital database that tracks the health and well-being of our two groups, offering the 10,000 enrollees in the second group any intervention, medical or nonmedical, that we believe will keep them healthy. If we know that X% of older adults forget to take their prescription medications and that this causes Y% to suffer acute health episodes requiring doctor visits or hospitalization, we buy everyone "smart" pill bottles that remind them to take their pills. Or, if we know that people who have hurt themselves in falls at home are less likely to fall at home again if the home is assessed for tripping hazards, we send someone to assess the home of anyone who has fallen, and then make changes accordingly. If one of the enrollees shows signs of malnourishment, we sign the person up with Meals on Wheels and also supply a digital scale that automatically reports his or her weight every morning to a central monitoring station. If someone is experiencing congestive heart failure, we monitor data on weight gain that indicates harmful fluid buildup and the need for a water-reduction pill. If the monitoring station does not receive satisfactory information on a particular aspect of a client's condition, a phone call or a home visit can be scheduled automatically. Even small changes from one day to the next can be captured and flagged for intervention before the problem produces a health crisis. If the intervention reduces a person's hospitalizations by 50%, we have spent a few hundred dollars on in-home devices but saved tens of thousands.

If, finally, in this scenario, we have access to a very large inventory of interventions, our 10,000 older adults will follow their natural inclination to seek the least medical, least invasive, least disruptive choices, according to the Law of Interchangeable Interventions. Because the interventions we offer are no longer confined within the boundaries of the medical sector, they will include options that a medical provider might not think about, such as a ride to the community center instead of antidepressant medication, or a half-hour visit three times a week from a physical therapist rather than pain medication and restricted activity, or a brief daily visit from a housekeeper instead of a move to assisted living for $300 per day. Plans of integrated care can adapt to new information immediately and continuously. Think of the program as an Interchangeable Interventions processor.

Given the growth of healthcare, finding less expensive alternatives is the best way society will be able to address the aging challenge. An enterprise will possess the data and tools to run control studies to compare the efficacy, costs, and safety among different possible interventions. That process will determine who does what. Data will guide decisions, not historical boundaries defined by disciplines or lobbyists.

If I am a business innovator who can combine my understanding of the Law of Interchangeable Interventions with my freedom from the constraints of the traditional healthcare sector, I can provide care for my population of 10,000 for much less than they now cost their various insurers. I can offer this less expensive care to the governor of a state that is responsible for 50% of the Medicaid cost for its citizens, a significant portion of whom are older and frail. Or, if that's too big a population for my new company to bite off right away, I can negotiate with a county executive whose local government is responsible for a share of the state's Medicaid costs. I can manage interventions flexibly rather than simply paying costs as treatments become necessary within the traditional medical sector. As is already the case with a few Medicaid benefits, I am not restricting health insurance coverage to medical expenses when lower-cost interventions can produce equivalent, or better, outcomes.

Such an outside-the-medical-box digital health insurer can coordinate drivers, homecare workers, telemedicine appointments, social workers, case managers, smart pills, and digital scales, just as Amazon did when it encouraged local entrepreneurs to build businesses that deliver packages under contract with Amazon. In the 21st-century digital economy, it isn't necessary to construct vast organizations from scratch to deliver goods or services. Pieces and programs can be linked. Data management and communications provide the glue that holds the pieces together, replacing the top-down command-and-control systems of the Industrial Age.

In present-day aging care, the networks are still primarily human. Two generations of a big family might be in and out of grandmother's house or apartment every day. She's never alone for long, and she's never left to forget to take her medications. In an alternative version of the story, the grandmother has no family nearby but lives on a street with longtime neighbors who work out a routine that, along with a paid household helper, keeps her safe and sound. In the coming world of aging care, in contrast, social interventions will be provided by housekeepers and visiting health providers who ride a small daily circuit of older adults' dwellings to provide beneficial interventions. These visitors act as professional daughters and sons who reproduce the loving family or caring neighborhood and help the older person stay home. Many of the caregivers don't need years of training. Unlike hospital care, with its billions of dollars of equipment, or time with a physician, the aging population can receive care from nonmedical staff. Workers will be abundantly available and can include neighborhood part-timers and gig workers. The technology that I have been describing does not replace human contact, but reduces the time needed for mechanical tasks, such as scheduling and route planning, and allows the caregivers to be patient and sympathetic. Freed from clerical tasks, caregivers will enjoy being able to engage in more fulfilling interactions with their clients.

What I'm sketching here, in short, is an approach to aging care that combines information management with the Law of Interchangeable Interventions. This exerts a natural downward pressure on spending. The lowering of costs, whether from replacing the specialist with the generalist or the medical with the social, has the beneficial effect of spreading consumer-preferred interventions more widely across communities. What will be created might be better titled *aging care insurance*, rather than medical insurance, with healthcare as one of its covered benefits.

A Model System: Digital Aging Care, Inc.

Let's create a model of this care system I've described for older people and see what it looks like. Let's call it Digital Aging Care, Inc., or DAC. In our model, DAC has a contract with a county to maintain, for a fixed fee per enrollee, the well-being and health of the county's population of dual-eligibles—those older adults who qualify for both Medicare (over 65), which covers hospital and medical expenses, and Medicaid (low income), which reimburses providers for custodial and support care. DAC has a database with extensive information on what keeps older people as healthy as is optimal for their age and conditions, or, to use my informal term, what keeps them in a State of Benescence. The database continuously collects, analyzes, and manages information from a wide range of sources to establish effective interventions for the ongoing changes in life circumstances a person encounters. Analysis of the information allows the system to recommend menus of interventions. DAC is notified by the system about a particular circumstance that might call for action, such as an ophthalmologist's report of diminished vision in an older adult who lives alone, and DAC also contracts with service providers who can carry out needed procedures and actions. DAC strives to coordinate many kinds of interventions, not merely medical ones, to maintain health.

Imagine that DAC learns from a client's smartphone records that he or she doesn't leave the apartment more than once or twice every 2 weeks. This information is matched with data about the client's health that indicates he or she is likely to benefit from group exercise sessions. The system searches the community for appropriate exercise opportunities and produces a plan including times, settings, transportation options, costs, required clothing or equipment, and an explanation of the expected benefits of joining an exercise program. A caseworker calls or visits with the older adult to discuss options and to make arrangements. What is unusual here is that the attention to the problem comes from the same company that follows the client's medical visits.

Now, let's imagine that the governor of a state recognizes that he or she is facing a financial budget crisis of monumental proportions, in large measure a result of the costs of providing care to older people. The cacophony of constantly inflating costs is simply overwhelming the state's other obligations. Constitutionally, the state cannot go into debt, unlike the federal government. One of the governor's policy advisers tells him or her about a looming technological behemoth, DAC, which would guarantee cost savings for the state of 30% within 2 years and 60% within 5 years, while promising greater customer satisfaction and guaranteeing safety. With no other options available, the governor agrees to meet with them.

The governor signs on. One month later, the governor calls DAC to say that there's a problem. The nurses' association has called complaining that their nurses are being displaced by aides who are now passing medications. DAC explains that control studies reflect that there is no reduction of safety with the specially trained aides. Nevertheless, the governor, feeling political pressure, requests that nurses return to the exclusive provision of this procedure. DAC agrees and informs the governor that the additional cost will be $7 per day for the unnecessary but requested additional nurse costs. Eventually, reduction of costs trumps political and previous historic practices, and the aides continue to pass medications safely and at less cost.

T.J.'s Story

T.J. lived all of his 86 years in his small Midwest town, historically an agricultural and manufacturing center. Over the past 20 years, agribusiness bought up the family farms and manufacturing disappeared. The kids moved away, leaving a residue of older men and women in limited economic circumstances. Things were bleak for T.J., who lost his job 25 years earlier when his manufacturing company moved to Mexico. He lived on Social Security, Medicaid, and Medicare. He survived two heart attacks and grappled with diabetes, renal failure, and chronic obstructive pulmonary disease from a lifetime of smoking. His activities were severely limited.

Then DAC came to town. Its community coordinator, in collaboration with the local aging council, set a goal to lower the healthcare premiums paid by the town citizens. DAC brought in experts to help the town select and develop programs they thought might be helpful. They began by offering a tax abatement to the local diner operator in exchange for adding healthy options to his menu. Discount coupons for the healthy options were distributed to people over 65. Eggs, oatmeal, decaffeinated coffee, and fresh orange juice were almost free. A group of older men gathered at the diner each morning, as they always had, but were now delighted to save money and began to eat more healthy choices instead of their usual donuts. Next door, tax incentives were extended to a grocer, and coupons for seniors were provided to encourage the purchase of fresh fruits and vegetables. The local church soup kitchen was also invited to purchase, at dramatic discounts, fresh fruits, vegetables, and dairy products. At the adjacent library, which was expanded by DAC, lectures, exercise, walking groups, tai chi, and yoga were introduced. A network among neighbors who signed up online was developed to help older adults share rides, prepare food, and look in on one another, all in order to encourage each other to improve their lives.

DAC arranged for T.J. to be picked up many mornings so that he could have breakfast at the diner with his friends of many years. Over time, he began to walk with the group before lunch. DAC coordinated all his needs and teamed him up with a neighbor to assure that he was in compliance with his care plan.

The local hospital had closed, and the nursing home had gone bankrupt. DAC contracted with a local nurse and a physical therapist to operate one remaining 12-unit wing of the old nursing home with an attached physical therapy room. DAC helped the town recruit a geriatric nurse practitioner by offering her a free house, a car, and rent-free office space (Doc Hollywood on steroids). Using the streamlined DAC charting and billing systems, she needed no experienced coding or *billing assistant. A telemedicine screen was set up so that some clients could talk to a regional physician situated two towns away. Periodically, an x-ray technician came to town to take x-rays, which were read on a screen 1,000 miles away. DAC made certain that T.J. became fully engaged with the clinic.*

One snowy afternoon, T.J. fell and broke his wrist. He was able to phone the clinic, which sent a neighbor to bring him in. There, the nurse gave him some pain medication and sent him in a neighbor's car to an orthopedist's office 120 miles away, where the bone was set. A few years later, despite T.J.'s involvement in better nutrition, exercise, and medication compliance, it became clear that he could no longer live at home alone. DAC was able to assure care in a small-scale group home. A widow with an older, substantial five-bedroom house received training to open a group home for people who needed meals and companionship. She also received a grant to install a stair glide and outside ramps, and to make bathroom renovations. There, T.J. was able to receive all the services DAC had been supplying in his home. The care was delivered at much less cost than would have been required if he had moved to a traditional nursing home. He remained as healthy as he would have been in that setting, but also remained with his life-long friends and in the community he had known for many years.

Next Steps

There is nothing in T.J.'s story that would require technologies that don't already exist. We still need to assemble a wide, aging care database that collects and sorts information from many sources. Selected information about the effectiveness of interventions in helping older adults to be in a State of Benescence will need to be collected, with the consent of the clients. The heart of the business will then be a database of interventions and providers crossed with a database of the results of the interventions that indicates what works best in a given set of circumstances. The inefficiencies and gaps in aging care as it exists today will attract technology companies from outside traditional healthcare to interconnect databases that already exist. Because we cannot afford to treat frailty in the upcoming generations with traditional healthcare methods, business will become eager to offer new solutions that will be profitable. Inevitably, entrepreneurs will be there to make money from new ways of delivering care. Because finding effective methods of supporting aging in place could yield a fortune, deep thinking, research, and investment will follow.

The central question of what interventions support successful aging in place isn't new, of course. Almost anyone approaching advanced age asks it, but there is a new urgency in the question as we look for ways to reduce the looming cost of aging care. The demographics will, at some point, win out. The massing of frailty and the industry's vestigial acute care orientation in the chronic era will overwhelm state budgets. State authorities will have no alternative but to hand over responsibility to entities that can operationalize the Law of Interchangeable Interventions and reset the momentum from spiraling costs and specialization. Such organizations will influence the historic scopes of practice guilds, once it is demonstrated that care interventions can be appropriately moved to other sectors of the economy. This sector convergence is occurring in virtually all other industries in the Digital Age. The only question is how much damage will occur to state budgets, societal resources, national competitiveness, and older adults before the bubble bursts and new-paradigm entities can form and rise to turn the tide.

If a company like DAC can capture the experiences of thousands of people concerning a particular intervention, such as transportation vouchers for rides to lunch at a community center or installing a telemedicine monitor at home, it can then match those experiences with individual profiles to determine which is the most appropriate choice at a particular moment. Ideally, DAC will supply interventions that are most likely to keep a person functioning at the same level today as he or she did yesterday.

Parallels to this already exist in our market economy, in the form of databases that collect information on the behaviors of large numbers of individuals in order to determine what any single individual is likely to purchase or how they will respond to an online ad. Algorithms monitor and manage transactions in many other very large systems, from retail (e.g., Amazon), to telecommunications (AT&T), to finance (MasterCard). Even the upcoming large numbers of older adults wouldn't cause a ripple in those systems. Amazon, for example, delivered 3.5 billion packages worldwide in 2019.[62] Using the same kind of information-gathering and management technology, we can collect data on what happens when we apply an intervention or a combination of interventions to thousands of people with wide ranges of conditions and needs. The mass of data that is now undifferentiated chaos to a traditional health insurer can be continuously analyzed, creating a dynamic, evolving health and wellness path. More people, more interventions, more failures and successes understood in ever-finer gradients of people's lives will allow more confident, more accurate, less invasive, and less expensive interventions. We just haven't done it yet.

The detailed information collected will provide a grasp of what would be most useful for each of DAC's individual enrollees. Contrast that with the nursing home I once operated where we treated everyone with essentially the same care regime, albeit with as much dignity and courtesy as we could manage. The fundamental hope is that using megadata to understand constantly changing conditions will give us more options and more individualization.

Some older adults among us have remained in a State of Benescence mostly on their own, perhaps with a little help from their family or friends. They have figured out by themselves how to age in place successfully. They go on living their lives as little disturbed as possible by changes in their physical capabilities, supported by interventions that are the least disruptive ones possible. They have been smart enough, lucky enough, or wealthy enough to find ways to achieve the safety and care of nursing homes without the frustrations and indignities of institutional life. The solutions they have found are models of the alternative we need to replace our traditional long-term care institutions, which are inadequate in size and cost for the new world of aging. Millions more people will have to age in place soon, and companies like DAC will make it possible for them to do so safely and appropriately.

Our present healthcare model, exemplified by Medicare and Medicaid, is like a car rental business with a large fleet that the owners never maintain, but only repair. They never change the oil in the cars and only open the hood when the engine overheats and stops. They need a very big repair shop (or hospital system). DAC, on the other hand, strives for more preventive maintenance and fewer breakdowns. This is hardly a revolutionary business idea, but it is not the way healthcare is organized today. In contrast, DAC will supply wraparound aging care management and health maintenance using a universe of interventions of which medicine is as small a part as possible. Maintaining people with nonmedical interventions will also produce a better quality of life than traditional medicalized healthcare. The demand will be large enough to attract large technology enterprises to compete for the business.

The population eligible for both Medicare and Medicaid, the dual-eligibles, is only about 20% of the total over-65 population. The other 80%, some 60 million people whose incomes are too high for Medicaid, are likely to develop the same care needs. They are subject to the same inevitable age-correlated losses of physical capacities and the same need to maintain a State of Benescence. If a largely nonmedical aging care regime works for some, it will work for many. If such a system keeps the dual-eligible Medicaid and Medicare recipient healthier, it will also be attractive as a health (or Benescence) option for the well insured and well-to-do. The digital technology–enabled future I see for aging gives preference to everything that supports and maintains health before it needs medical interventions. Medical care will come as a last resort when nothing else would be as effective. Anyone, rich or poor, can benefit from the working of the Law of Interchangeable Interventions.

As described previously, Medicare-only clients receive coverage for medical-based care only and have no coverage for custodial or supportive care. This may seem to leave DAC out of the action for the Medicare population, given that so much of what DAC supplies is not medical. But what if the Center for Medicare and Medicaid Services, the federal agency that administers both programs, could be persuaded of the advantages to their budgets of the Law of Interchangeable Interventions? If they became convinced that offering nonmedical interventions could reduce the cost of medical interventions, a sea change in aging care and its costs would result.

In 2017, people eligible for both Medicare and Medicaid accounted for approximately $423 billion in federal and state spending by these agencies. Walmart, the largest corporation in the United States by revenue, took in $486 billion in the same year.[63] If DAC were supplying everything the dual-eligible population was buying for healthcare, it would have a business about the size of Walmart's. The population of poor older adults constitutes an enormous market.

Combining Big Data and a Multidisciplinary Team

Let's stop for a moment and take a closer look at how a company like DAC works. The previous pages described the services it will be providing, but it is also worth taking a look into the organization itself, and to see how it will approach a new community that awards it a contract.

Accumulating big data as I have described is critical and necessary, but by itself it is insufficient. It is true that for a 92-year-old with eight chronic conditions, big data can utilize constant feedback to determine risk factors and suggest interventions that reduce further losses. But while computer algorithms may help to elucidate what is happening, a well-trained multidisciplinary team of people utilizing the digital analyses will pinpoint the unfolding dynamics and set in motion the best approaches to mitigate damage and recapture capabilities. Responding quickly can be the difference between life and death, between years of robust health and diminished living. The ongoing accumulation of data uncovers what to the naked eye may appear as a stable state but is actually a very complex dynamic. So, rather than eliminating the human element, big data may open a need for even more sophisticated human decision making.

How does DAC operationalize the required combination of big data with a multidisciplinary team? Imagine that in an area of 1 million inhabitants, 37,000 dual-eligibles live, many of them frail.* They request the services of DAC. The company selects a seasoned leader from another, well-established DAC team to build the new initiative. The primary role of the leader is to create and empower a team to make decisions. Together with other veteran DAC participants, the leader carefully recruits a local team of nine established professionals:

---

*In 2018, there were 12.2 million dual-eligibles in a population of 330 million Americans (Data Analysis Brief: Medicare-Medicaid Dual Enrollment 2006 through 2018. https://www. cms.gov/Medicare-Medicaid-Coordination/Medicare-and-Medicaid-Coordination/Medicare-Medicaid-Coordination-Office/DataStatisticalResources/Downloads/MedicareMedicaidDual EnrollmentEverEnrolledTrendsDataBrief2006-2018.pdf).

- Social worker
- Nurse
- Therapist
- Geriatrician
- Community liaison
- Digital analyst
- Digital programmer
- Licensed homecare aide
- Budget analyst

Each has extensive professional expertise and proven sensitivity to older adults. Team orientation, a trusting nature, and curiosity are also critical traits, as is a predisposition to reach out to other disciplines and span traditional boundaries.

The team members sequester together in an intensive 6-week team-building training program. The focus is on the DAC mission, which is ensuring the safety, happiness, and health of the clients. This organizational mantra remains central throughout the training. The first part of the orientation comprises physical challenges requiring the team to rely on one another. The other two-thirds of the time consists of extensive participatory decision-making simulations that force team members to listen to one another, to weigh and balance their different perspectives, and to come to shared decisions regarding proper interventions. Using the techniques and language of creative problem solving, exercises are designed on the DAC big data network where the team learns to integrate the information with the tools available.

The simulations start rather simply and then begin adding more variables, such as the dollar cost of each intervention, determining camera and sensor locations for data collection in particular clients' dwellings, and the coordination of socialization interventions such as the benefits of engaging neighbors to spend time with a client. The team then discusses and critiques each decision, evaluating what it had not weighed fully or had missed altogether. The exercises demonstrate how choices based on only one or two disciplines often have less beneficial results than more nuanced, multidisciplinary ones. The exercises become increasingly complex, with tighter time constraints. The consequences of the decisions are analyzed and compared with the consequences of alternative paths not taken.

One day each week the team travels together to a neighboring, fully functioning DAC team site. Each team member is buddied with the corresponding person of his or her own discipline. The mornings demonstrate the workings of the host team as a unit. In the afternoon, visiting team members shadow a person from a different discipline. The pairs rotate so that at the end of 6 weeks, each team member has been able to view the system from a variety of different perspectives. Every week, each team member makes a full report of both parts of the visit.

Funding Sources

How does DAC acquire the resources to train and support such a skilled team? This question goes to the heart of the company. First, DAC produces a savings from not using institutional care, as well as by replacing more expensive surgeries with medicine and more expensive medicine with social interventions, whenever it is possible to do so without reducing effectiveness for the client. Maintaining people in their existing community homes and apartments eliminates the cost of specialized physical plants. These are the most dramatic savings, and they are accompanied by a series of carefully designed features in the DAC team structure.

Historically, there have been few cost comparisons among different categories of interventions paid for by Medicare. As long as an intervention fits within a given Medicare category, higher costs are passed on to the government with few questions asked. No one presses for lower costs. Dollars simply float up to more expensive specialists and procedures. Therefore, there has been no incentive to shift costs into preventive measures that save higher expenses from occurring. Providers have not been trained or incentivized to do so, nor do they have readily available access to information that would enable them to prevent dramatic, invasive interventions. DAC, on the other hand, will be motivated to invest in interventions that avoid and reduce expensive procedures because the company will directly benefit from the savings. These reductions, combined with the savings from deinstitutionalization, will allow DAC to function at a much lower cost per person.

Reducing expenses is an essential purpose of the DAC's locally embedded teams. Each team has the range of skill sets to evaluate the most appropriate, safe, and inexpensive approaches, both short- and long-term. With access to the full range of social, medical, and surgical interventions rather than the narrower range of only medical options, team members have the means to find savings throughout the decision-making process.

The team's procedures are created to capture efficiencies that are not possible in the traditional delivery system for aging. First, DAC's digital network has automatically collected, sorted, and analyzed much of the critical information that previously dominated staff time. Second, it reduces and speeds up the decision-making process of the team. Historically, individuals or lower-level teams make recommendations that are passed up the chain of command until they reach the person with the full scope of authority to make a decision. The initial recommendation is always at risk for delayed or faulty decisions by people far from the frontlines. In contrast, the DAC team has all of the relevant facts and implications of a case to make a decision. It does not need to send a memo or an envoy to cajole, convince, or explain the recommendation.

Traditional large-scale aging institutions like nursing homes use economies of scale to deliver care. This requires middle management to set up ironclad systems for basic caregivers' routines. At DAC, Industrial Age departments such as human resources or the business office are incorporated into the team's function or are decreased. The DAC team leader evaluates the effectiveness of each team member rather than passing the task to a human resources executive. The regional supervisor helps to counsel or replace a floundering member. The regional supervisor analyzes and makes changes to teams that are not functioning effectively. Much of the traditional business office functions, such as the evaluation of the expenses against budget, are absorbed into the daily decisions of the DAC team. And because the DAC is itself the health insurer, teams have less need to negotiate with outsiders for approvals regarding reimbursement for their decisions. Computer algorithms already incorporate state and federal regulations, so decisions can be made with minimal holdup for outside approvals.

Savings go even further because of the team structure. It minimizes the need for in-service programs that regularly remove low-wage workers from their tasks and gather them together for training. At DAC, continuing education is integrated on an ongoing basis into computer updates and the networking process. When the system suggests an intervention, the computer will search for availability and price, and it will also rank local programs and interventions for effectiveness depending on an individual's particular requirements. Because the interventions and algorithms are based on large control-group studies and on comparisons with results in thousands of similar cases, there is less need for additional evaluation.

Some of the savings from all these new procedures go into digital network capacity, where, once installed, programs can be used indefinitely for minimal additional cost. Savings are also invested in the salaries of team members, which enables DAC to hire and hold the best and the brightest. In the Industrial Age delivery system, enormous resources are siphoned off from caregiving and devoted to highly paid executives, as well as middle managers who operate centralized departments such as dietary, human resources, and building acquisition. Many of these expenses can be reduced by an organization like DAC. Uber, Airbnb, and some large banks have realized similar savings.

If one assumes that government will not have the funds to significantly increase Medicare and Medicaid rates, the only realistic way to increase wages is to cut existing costs from within the system. By lifting many of the frustrating constraints that impede staff in Industrial Age organizations for aging, DAC team members are able to devote their time and skills to helping older adults directly and to creating a stimulating, supportive, exciting environment for them.

The DAC network is constantly updated with data from the community and providers. Team leaders as well as team members attend weekly video meetings with their discipline counterparts from other DAC sites to discuss new findings and challenges that they bring back to their local team. Updates to the algorithms are regularly transmitted to the team for discussion and inclusion. Once a month, each team member embeds for a day in a different DAC site, constantly cross-pollinating ideas and approaches. The result is a team of teams. Because the entire team has access to so much information on their computers and phones, they can provide constant and consistent support. In order to participate, contractors and subcontractors must spend time at the DAC site. They learn the DAC software so that their input and reports become an essential core of their work. Providers and potential providers support the DAC culture, focusing on participant safety, happiness, and health.

The roles of the specific team members, and even their titles, reflect the values of DAC. For example, rather than a business manager, the team includes a dollar analyst, whose role is to embed expenditures within the algorithms and interventions so the team can manage expenditures and investments in the most prudent manner. The expenditures per person, category, and provider are calculated in real time for all DAC team members. The team can develop an informed approach to the full arc of a challenge. With the data, the team can consider the unique circumstances of a person with a hip fracture and forecast an entire rehabilitation process, weighing the relative effectiveness of alternative pathways as they present themselves. These factors and outcomes can be benchmarked against the experience of other teams locally and around the state.

Geriatricians discover that, through DAC, they finally have an organizational base that supports their training as coordinators and leaders of both medical and nonmedical services. Because the goal is to catch changes in and threats to participant's well-being as soon as possible, geriatricians teach the entire workforce what to watch for and when to signal presenting issues for medical review.

The Industrial Age's healthcare system of creating specialized silos has framed the entire delivery system for older people. The treatment of mental health, for example, was split off from physical health. As a result, "health professionals . . . have treated mind and body differently and cared for them under different systems."[64] Poor integration between the two systems creates major challenges in meeting the complex needs of adults with severe mental illness. They often have difficulties obtaining general healthcare. This is particularly unfortunate, for those individuals tend to have higher rates of chronic general medical conditions.[65]

Even within the category of behavioral health, separate silos often present overwhelming barriers to appropriate care. For example, in 2021, "the number of yearly overdose fatalities surpassed 100,000."[66] Yet in many states the addiction-treatment system is separate from the mental health system, and each system may be prohibited from treating a condition unless it is the primary diagnosis. The systems "treat people who suffer from both mental health and substance abuse disorders as the exception, when in fact they are the rule."[67] Even when both systems are accessible, their interventions may be at odds with one another. For many, care is "haphazard—uncoordinated and disconnected from (a person's) actual needs."[68]

The DAC team-centered culture moves staff away from the traditional silos-by-discipline of Industrial Age institutions, where energy is wasted on battles between departments for resources. Because DAC engages the full range of institutions and community providers, incorporating them into a fluid network of ongoing interactions, the locked-down constraints give way. Although the particular knowledge of a discipline is a critical competency for a DAC team member, what comes to the fore is each person's capacity to engage productively with the other disciplines. Each professional has obligations to his or her discipline, to the standards in his or her license, and to DAC.

New career opportunities will arise for many trained professionals. Historically, career ladders have been locked down, restricted within one's discipline. Some therapists, nurses, and social workers excel at their crafts, yet can become frustrated by the tedium after 10 or 20 years. They may hold enormous untapped management and leadership capacities that will flourish at DAC. The team-oriented organizational structure enables extended skills and leadership abilities to emerge. Staff can learn on the job, finding and developing talent to meet new opportunities. All along the previous restricted scopes of certain practices, professionals will be relieved of chores that others can do more efficiently, and can then assume responsibilities for tasks that more accurately match their full capabilities and experience. The most highly trained health professionals will no longer be tethered to tasks that they are currently required to carry out but will be free to explore and invent new methods of aging care. Emotional resistance to the dramatic changes in each historic scope of practice will be overcome by making responsibilities for each more stimulating and exciting. Professionals will no longer practice at the top of their license but at the top of their imagination and ability.

Depending on the resources of the community, both the initial composition of the team and its changing shape will evolve. The available labor for homecare or geriatricians may vary widely in different locales, as may the need for particular kinds of care. DAC collects variations of human resource patterns from DAC sites around the country and suggests organizational frameworks to fit the locale. For example, DAC teams may scale up or down the number of social workers for ongoing contact with clients, or they may utilize people from other disciplines with the necessary skill sets.

Critical to DAC's success is rapid yet safe innovation as new interventions are developed. This necessitates thousands of small-scale trials. Regulators are embedded in the DAC team network and involved in the initial development of control studies. They confer with corresponding regulators in other locales to evaluate the reliability and validity of the results and to approve successful innovations. These are shared throughout the DAC network. New checklists, while critical, are not followed as ironclad rules. Rather, they are appended to the innovation as suggested "how-to's" to be considered and perhaps adapted by a local team.

The staff member designated as the community liaison brings the entire local community into the enterprise of caring for its older adults. This person is not a community developer or organizer, for the outside community already exists. Nor is he or she developing the community around the DAC organization. This person's role is to tie them together. The activities of some existing community service organizations may expand or combine. For example, Meals on Wheels and its corps of volunteers can report on a host of factors regarding the status of each client. Grocery chains, restaurants, food pantries, and senior center nutrition sites can be integrated to ensure food security. As DAC matures, it may engage a volunteer group to retrieve and recondition assistive devices such as wheelchairs, walkers, crutches, and canes when people outgrow them, so that they can be reused by others.

DAC dramatically extends both the reach and breadth of traditional PACE programs. No longer obligated to bring clients to a physical day center, it uses digital technology to engage and evaluate participants while they remain in their homes in the community. It extends its services to all older adults, not merely the most frail. And DAC is scalable to very large populations through its ability to insert small teams wherever necessary. Whereas PACE programs are boutiques, with their operations centered very precisely around a small cadre of people, DAC is open ended, with the potential to care flexibly for millions. The digitization and computer analysis of data allows responses to be immediate. This eliminates much of the time and energy searching for and collating data in order to make decisions.

DAC is also a quantum leap over the Town Square framework that I attempted to develop, described in Chapter 7. My original idea used physical co-location to coordinate a range of pre-existing disparate community-based agencies. None of the Town Square agencies had the resources or expertise to extend the services to a frail population of the size of the one that formerly resided in nursing homes and now needs care in their homes. The agencies I worked with were tied to existing, albeit inadequate, funding streams and organizational boundaries. They did not have the resources or residual energy to invest in a new, very different venture. The Town Square also had no ability to communicate and coordinate services with its other agencies or to allocate revenues among themselves easily. In contrast, DAC is a cross-disciplinary organization without the distractions of multiple masters, disparate regulations, and funding sources. Nor is it confronted with the near-impossible task of coordinating interventions and allocating reimbursements among different agencies.

DAC is designed to utilize the Law of Interchangeable Interventions. It dramatically expands and extends the healthcare delivery system. The current acute care–oriented system is focused on more dramatic interventions, so it has ignored entire areas of research. There has been little interest in and minimal financial support for such fields as social gerontology and public health for older adults. By analyzing the entire aging ecosystem for compounding risks and exploring the full palette of possible interventions, DAC creates opportunities, supported by funding from the health system, to invest in the full range of social, nonmedical components of a population's health.

There are untapped disciplines waiting to be mined for opportunities to head off and mitigate the burdensome costs of frailty in older age. Under our current system, we pay the bill in the hospital, but the actual costs come from what has happened before we ever got there. This is no different from going to a restaurant and enjoying a feast with a whole family. The cost is really from the preparation of the food in the kitchen, not the service at the table. We ignore frailty while it festers in the community, where the real costs accumulate, leaving it unattended until it ripens into a full-blown crisis. After a hospital stay costing thousands of dollars, a person is stabilized and returned to a community that cannot support him or her, and the cycle begins again. DAC introduces a finely tuned, population-based health system that integrates social and medical interventions oriented toward prevention and mitigation, as well as cure. It keeps costs down, and the meal tastes even better.

Is DAC, which is, after all, a fictional company, really possible? Can our present healthcare system, an Industrial Age behemoth, be adapted to address this enormous new challenge? Gen. Stanley McChrystal, in *Team of Teams*,[69] described how our highly regimented armed forces were decentralized into small adaptive teams, using emergent intelligence to defeat a constantly changing enemy in Iraq; how General Motors survived by quickly restructuring itself into "team-like oneness across an enterprise of ten thousand,"[70] and how NASA used adaptive, emergent intelligence to escape from constant failure to develop the Apollo project, described by Robert Seamans and Frederick Ordway as "generally considered one of the greatest technological endeavors in the history of mankind."[71] Throughout the United States, corporate leadership has dramatically improved productivity through small-group decision-making connected through neural networks.[72] As McChrystal's examples indicate, elements of all the suggested DAC team operations already exist or can be adapted from programs that exist elsewhere. It may be difficult to believe that small-scale, embedded teams can replace the mighty citadels of the Industrial Age healthcare system in the Digital Age, but they can, and they will. The next chapter will explore further some of the challenges and changes that this transition will face.

The Special Case of Dementia

Dementia is a particular condition that cannot be handled in the same way as many of the chronic conditions of growing older. It occupies a unique place in the world of aging and care. Various types of dementia, especially Alzheimer's disease, have gained new prominence as longevity has increased. Dementia is highly correlated with age, although it is not inherent in aging itself. Because the number of older adults is increasing, annual cases of dementia are expected to double in 30 years. By 2050, when the U.S. population is projected to be 438 million, the number of people over 65 with dementia may grow from 5.5 million (in 2017) to 13.8 million (in 2060). Half of the individuals with dementia will be over 85.[73] They will be a significant factor in planning to care for older people and will require care that is different from care for individuals with other kinds of chronic conditions that we have been discussing in this volume.

Dementia is now understood to be a disease of very long duration, in which the neurons of the brain are degenerating. The average duration of the disease from onset is thought to be 10 years.[74] Even the diagnosis itself is difficult, and it is often hard to distinguish one type of dementia from another. Neurologists attempt to rule out other treatable conditions, such as depression or drug interactions. Although effective drug interventions do not exist currently, there is new thinking that "there are nine risk factors accounting for much of the world's dementia: high blood pressure, lower education levels, impaired hearing, smoking, obesity, depression, physical inactivity, diabetes, and low levels of social contact . . . researchers estimated about 62 percent of current dementia cases could have been prevented across risk factors."[75] Unfortunately, although many of these factors can be approached within the community, our primary focus remains on pharmaceutical options.

So far, there's very little we can do to change the progression once dementia is diagnosed. Compared to all the progress with cardiovascular issues and cancer, as well as more recent developments in genomics, we remain stumped about brain disorders. Ironically, even though President George H. W. Bush designated the 1990s as the "decade of the brain," we have not been able to unlock the mysteries of major cognitive disorders. There is some thinking that Alzheimer's is "(not) primarily a disease of the brain . . . but rather . . . a disorder of the immune system within the brain."[76] Whether it is a disease, a combination of diseases and chronic conditions, or an autoimmune disease, dementia is currently outside the realm of significant medical intervention.

Even the recognition of dementia as a disease did not bring new interventions and resources to bear, as medical research has done for some other age-correlated conditions. Paradoxically, our traditional healthcare delivery platforms are moving away from, rather than toward, the dementia challenge. As nursing homes move from the long-term custodial care of Medicaid clients to shorter-term Medicare clients, the reimbursement system pushes facilities to favor admitting people with physical limitations. People with dementia, however, often retain physical capabilities until very late in the disease progression. The costs of surveillance and care, even for people with mid-stage dementia, are significant, but the amount of nursing home reimbursement for which they qualify is insufficient. In many states, dementia has been effectively excised from the health system, including the mental health sector.

Even before nursing homes were not as medicalized as they have become, their traditional physical and programmatic template was not appropriate for dementia. Their programmatic design focused on nursing, medications, and treatments that are often not useful for many people with early and mid-stage memory loss. The standard two-person bedrooms created ongoing difficulties with roommates. The traditional building design provided insufficient recreation space. Residents with dementia may have to be kept in close proximity to nursing stations for surveillance, creating a need to restrain them with psychotropic medications or Geri-chairs, all the while coordinating with the health department's shifting definitions and prohibitions around restraints. Many of the difficult behaviors associated with dementia are created or exacerbated by a nursing home's design. For example, a person's inability to move away or verbalize discomforts when others crowd them can result in a reaction that may be interpreted as acting out.

The nub of the dementia challenge is tied to the underlying problem of inappropriately placing people requiring chronic care into medicalized settings. In many of our traditional settings, tasks around medicalization push out social interventions that are appropriate for dementia-related constellations of symptoms. The person with memory loss often remains frozen in the kind of system that dominated the mid-20th century, when there were few beneficial interventions for any person, and nursing homes were more custodial than medical. Yet, historically, those nursing homes have been the only available places to house the person safely.

More recently, memory care units in assisted-living communities have become an option for people with dementia. These purpose-built environments for dementia are designed to address the nature of the condition. They have a less institutionalized design, with settings that facilitate flexible socializing, eating, toileting, bathing, and sleeping. Caregivers are oriented to understand the nature of dementia and armed with the skills to head off and diffuse tensions. Such memory care units, however, are not economically accessible to the majority of older adults.

As the medicalization of nursing homes renders them increasingly inappropriate for people with dementia, more affected individuals live at home in their communities for years. Moreover, a person with memory loss is unable to communicate his or her needs in order to avail him- or herself of the benefits of the Law of Interchangeable Interventions. This has often resulted in a disastrous emotional, physical, and financial toll on families.

Because so many people with dementia remain in the community, it is critical that interventions be developed for use in their residences. Home environments need adaptation to the unique nature of memory impairment, with cues to help the older adult navigate and safety proofing to avoid injury. Internal door locks must be fixed so that the person with dementia doesn't get locked in by accident and for a partner to be able to separate him- or herself for protection. There must be a hotline so that the partner can call someone who has working knowledge of the situation and can provide guidance and support. People need homecare to arrive quickly if necessary, either with medication or to provide safety.

The looming scale and challenges of memory loss are evidenced in Japan, the nation with the world's oldest population. Currently, people with dementia constitute about 4.3% of their population, and some predict that by 2045, 20% will have the condition.[77] Because the numbers are already beyond many communities' ability to house people in special-built facilities, older men and women remain in home environments from which they frequently abscond into the community. A few communities have developed extensive digital tracking systems. Itami, a suburb of Osaka, has installed more than

1,000 sensors that line the streets. Tracking devices can be placed on the person to locate and send messages to family members. Issues around privacy, loss of dignity, and informal consent, however, have dramatically limited the registration of older adults. Ironically, nearly half of all elementary students were registered.[77]

There are some signs that the nature and scale of the dementia challenge is beginning to be addressed in the United States. Historically closed off from being adequately addressed in our healthcare system, dementia will eventually find itself accommodated in the same venue as other age-correlated chronic conditions: the community. A prototype can be found in Dementia Friendly America, a national movement that coalesced in 2015 following a White House conference on aging. It is a network of communities that equip themselves with education, skills, and programs to enable people with dementia to be retained in their midst. It may be a forerunner, similar to early senior centers, of a community-based movement that reformats care from a medical base with a light sprinkling of social support to one with a social foundation where medical interventions are available and dropped in as appropriate.

Conclusion

I believe digital technology will change the experience of getting older at the local and individual level by allowing us to aggregate and understand the experiences of aging at a global level. As programs collect data and analyze more and more about the full, multidimensional aging experience, more and more opportunities to help almost any individual will appear. We can benefit enormously from the collected experience of the older population. The life lived on a particular block will reap the benefits of the experiences of the later years of life everywhere. Until now, we lived and aged in particular places with local and personal circumstances; digital technology will allow us to live locally and, at the same time, to draw from the greater community of everyone else who is adding on years. We will still be our individual aging selves but informed by the wisdom and experience of the entire universe of people growing older.

CHAPTER 13

The New World of Aging

When I was young, I spent many of my summers in upstate Wisconsin. At age 10 or so, I remember evenings wandering alone around a swamp, exploring the swamp gas, the sticky, soft, warm water's edge, the sounds of bullfrogs, the blue dragonflies that seemed to fly sideways like helicopters. I would pick up large stones over my head and dump them in the deep silent pool, *kerplunk*. The stone disappeared, there was a long hesitation, and then came a deep sound like an explosion, followed by an eruption of water, in my mind like a cannonball in slow motion. I also remember dreamily picking up flat stones for skipping along the water's surface. Or I grabbed handfuls of pebbles, heaving them into the pond and watching as they formed a slow pattern of blips and then coalesced and created wonderful patterns on the surface.

A Vision of the Future of Aging

The future of aging is not the "kerplunk" of one huge stone, even though it is true that a population and longevity tsunami is coming. Nor is aging's future like skipping or gliding stones over the surface of the pond, with minimal impact and hardly a sound. The change in aging is more like throwing handfuls of various components into the mix and watching them interact. Demographics, economics, reimbursements, institutions, regulations, labor forces, technology, and science are all sent into a swirl. The resulting pattern of each toss has its own character, history, posture, and trajectory. If we find some patterns in their interactions, we can come to a deeper understanding of what is happening and how the future could unfold in my optimistic and hypothetical new world of aging, liberated from physical and institutional constraints. We had a taste of Mrs. Smith's potential lifestyle in the Introduction as well as descriptions of the hypothetical clients served by Digital Aging Care, Inc. (DAC), in Chapter 12. When we combine a new and more realistic understanding of aging in the 21st century with the advantages of digital technology, and allow the Law of Interchangeable Interventions to work without too many restrictions, we will see wonderful new patterns forming wherever we turn.

As described in the previous chapters of this book, we are anxious about getting older in great part because of what we have seen and known of 20th-century aging. Our impressions have been formed by what we know from witnessing the medicalization and institutionalization of aging care in the past 75 years. Traditional-style hospitals and nursing homes figure prominently in our mental pictures. Attempts to change the landscape have produced assisted living and memory care facilities, senior apartment houses, retirement communities, and other arrangements, but these continue to segregate older adults from the everyday life of communities. Our sense of dread about aging is amplified by the slowly dawning realization that the aging population is exploding to enormous numbers that our present system does not have the resources to care for. All we can see is a future with sicker and sicker older people filling hospitals, nursing homes, and assisted living situations until there is no more room or money. Even if we read or hear that older age can be filled with insight and experience, our picture of those years is usually still one of poor health and decline.

In the next 20 years, we will see a revolution in the toolbox of integrated interventions for older adults that will improve the functional status of both individuals and the wider population. The new options will radically reduce the expense of healthcare services for our oldest age cohort. This won't be a revolution in medicine, although there will be breakthroughs, but in other kinds of interventions. The care model I proposed with the hypothetical DAC is not part of the medical care system. Today's idea of aging care, subservient to the medical system, is still much too passive with respect to maintaining a person in a State of Benescence, even though it is aggressive when ill health requires medical care. What I project for the future of aging care will be just as aggressive about supplementing and maintaining individual capacity with every possible kind of support, including medicine when appropriate. Each client will have a care manager, who orchestrates the work of the subcontractors who provide services ranging from grocery delivery and home surveillance to transportation and home medical treatments. The care manager will use the digital environment around each enrollee to coordinate interventions, always with the goal of keeping enrollees on an even keel. The digital environment will include the continuous monitoring by automatic data collection of physical, emotional, social, and environmental markers of well-being, as well as the continuous evaluation of that data to signal if a review is needed. This environment extends to everyone the aging care–related benefits that are now accessed only by the wealthy who can afford wide-ranging private services.

As described in Chapter 12, what took manpower before, and was therefore relatively expensive, will now use computing power, accumulate data much more quickly, allow for more refined information, and cost much less. If DAC gives everyone under its umbrella the advantages now enjoyed by the wealthy, then everyone can be as healthy as the top few percent are today. Everyone will be in included in the same wide networks of data. In this future world, everyone, rich and poor, lives better. Continuous management of chronic conditions will eliminate or mitigate many of the episodes that now limit people's capacities and activities and often put them in the hospital, where they are in great danger of suffering complications. Operating according to the Law of Interchangeable Interventions, it will reduce the need for the kind of healthcare that hospitals provide today.

At the risk of repetition, let me give one more example of how a client's experience might go, emphasizing the reduced role of traditional medical care when DAC determines the best possible options.

Oliver's Story

At 96, since his beloved spouse died 10 years ago, Oliver continued to live comfortably in his house of 60 years. His daughter, Suzanne, lived 25 minutes away and remained intimately involved without devoting an undue amount of time to his needs. In fact, she was able to retain her role as doting daughter rather than as a full-time caregiver or care coordinator.

Some time ago, under DAC's supervision, Oliver moved his bed down to the first-floor den, and the adjacent half-bathroom was expanded appropriately. Despite Oliver's five chronic conditions, he was happy to have the interventions that enabled him to remain in a State of Benescence. Oliver awakened each morning and used a toilet that spritzed and air-dried his bottom. He brushed his hair and teeth, stood on the scale, donned a robe, and walked to the kitchen. He was already hooked into his support system. His weight was transmitted to a database and compared to his previous weights. The toilet analyzed his urine. Cameras captured and evaluated his gait for unsteadiness.

By hooking up to his phone, readings of his blood pressure and blood chemistry were transmitted, as were readings from his pacemaker, defibrillator, and internal insulin pump. An adjustment was recommended, Oliver and his daughter were notified, and new medications were delivered through the wall delivery panel of his front door later that morning. The daily aide took in the new meds and rearranged Oliver's pill box according to the updated medical chart on her phone. Every few months, perhaps, a nurse came in early, before Oliver was dressed, and took pictures that were read 1,000 miles away for signs of skin cancer.

As Oliver lost and gained capabilities with various activities of daily living, such as continence, dressing, or medication compliance, changes were prescribed on the aide's phone, and small adjustments were made immediately. Damp diapers sent the aide a signal, and chips in each pill signaled when it hit the digestive tract and could provide accurate blood chemistry readings.

Breakfast was easy, as were other meals and even snacks. Coffee was started by voice command. Oliver ordered food through a computer program that took into account his nutritional needs, allergies, preferences, and ability to prepare it. The food was delivered directly into his fridge through the wall unit on his porch.

The timing and necessary qualifications of caregivers were constantly updated, balanced, and adjusted according to Oliver's changing needs, with the goal of keeping care and costs to a minimum. The care plan was a clear, integrated set of directives. All the caregivers carried interactive schedules that adjusted locations, duties, and routines in real time. They negotiated their employment rates with Suzanne, and their performance was evaluated. Access to Oliver's home was by fingerprint identification, matched to the individual caregiver's schedule.

Oliver was delighted to remain at home, even though his daughter was initially concerned that, housebound and without social stimulation, he would become bored, reclusive, and depressed. However, the same network system that coordinated his physical care *also kept him engaged in activities of various kinds. His multichannel television with enhanced sound fed directly into his hearing aid and included video for streaming lectures and discussions, where he could see the other participants. It was almost a senior center at home. Oliver could also sign up online to attend any number of community events in person. Transportation was scheduled, and an aide arrived to prepare him so that his daughter did not have to orchestrate the activity. Even alone at home, Oliver's interests and patterns were stimulated. A pleasant voice gently suggested to Oliver that he watch favorite programs, call friends at an accustomed time, or take a walk. His choices were tracked to refine future suggestions.*

When Oliver fell, he was unable to call for help, but his wrist phone captured his unconscious state and called an ambulance that was given access to his locked door. The EMTs could call up his care plan, as did the hospital upon his arrival. His daughter was automatically notified to meet him at the emergency department and, in conference with the doctor and the care manager, decided that Oliver would undergo hip replacement surgery. After 3 days, Oliver went to a rehab center where he was carefully monitored during physical therapy. Four days later, he returned home where a new bed and wheelchair were awaiting him, as were his new meds, care plan, therapy program, and aides who had been selected to meet his changed needs. The food delivered to his home reflected his post-op status, as well as his preferences. For the first week, food deliveries were followed by a very careful scrutiny of both intake and output.

A few years later, Oliver began to become confused. Cameras were set up to monitor him. Doors and kitchen equipment were programmed to open or lock to assure his safety. His food was adjusted to include more items that were easy to prepare and eat. Staffing shifted to aides trained in dementia care. Local neighbors, who had submitted their names to a digital bulletin board and were screened by Oliver's daughter, were paid to sit with him from time to time. During those years of confusion, Oliver was a candidate for dementia day care. His care manager had access to all such programs in the area, with information about their availability, the range of clients in their care, the training of the staff, ratings for each program, and the costs. Accompanied by a dementia specialist, Suzanne visited the top three programs and selected the most promising. At first, Oliver

attended 3 days a week, and he eventually increased that to 5 days.
Aides arrived at his home in the morning to prepare him for pick up.
The vehicle, its driver, and an attendant were all selected to conform
to Oliver's mobility and behavioral risks.

Oliver eventually lost his ability to speak and to walk. The pallia-
tive care unit adapted his environment, food, equipment, staffing, and
medications to his bed-bound circumstances. He developed an infec-
tion, was kept comfortable, and died at home. In all these years, Oliver
spent no more than a few days in a nursing home, and he maintained
a comfortable State of Benescence.

Developing the Model

There will certainly be obstacles to overcome in developing my model
for the future, including worries about privacy, as discussed previously.
The new system depends on a mega-database that is programmed to
make multiple kinds of connections between information *from* enrollees and information *for* enrollees. This super network will need to be
assembled. Collecting the results of millions of interventions as well
as additional data from tens of millions of Americans, not to mention
adapting existing algorithms and writing new ones, will all require
an initial investment. The technology exists, but creating the overall
orchestrating program will require billions of dollars.

A similar problem presented itself during the development of
radio. In *One Summer: America 1927*, Bill Bryson explained that the
science that enabled the immediate transmission from voices far
away was miraculous, but people were not buying radios because
there was minimal content to listen to. Program development costs
were staggeringly expensive. The answer the broadcasting companies found was advertising. Companies would pay to induce people
to buy their wares, and listeners didn't mind.[78]

For DAC, the cost of developing integrated content through writing code, licensing, joint venturing, and merging with other entities can
eventually be paid for from funds already being collected from clients
of Medicare and Medicaid. DAC will also find private investors who
have confidence that government will be eager to sign up. Once people
begin to understand the seismic change in growing old that DAC ush-
ers in, participants will multiply. Eventually, a few large management

corporations using digital tools will be able to reach a sustainable level of surplus while keeping older and frail people healthy at home for much less than we spend now and with better results.

Along the way, organizations like DAC will need to address a whole range of marketing, technological, labor, and regulatory challenges. In time, a new network paradigm will overtake an enormous, historically mature industry. There are such potential benefits to be achieved, and such high profits to be made, that the new approach will infiltrate and replace the old. I believe it will occur quickly when the time is ripe. And with aging, the time is ripe.

The New Model Reshapes Traditional Healthcare as We Have Known It

Let's investigate how some parts of the new system will look under the new paradigm.

Insurance

In its title, "How Did Healthcare Get to Be Such a Mess?"[79] historian Christy Ford Chapin's *New York Times* article served up the fundamental question regarding our healthcare system. Her book, *Ensuring America's Health,*[80] laid out the unrecognized history of the healthcare system in the United States. It resulted in an idiosyncratic but powerful system that is so deep and unshakable that it renders ineffectual many attempts to reshape it.

The concept of private health insurance, now firmly embedded in thinking about healthcare in the United States, was not preordained. As medical care was evolving in the 20th century, there were multiple alternative approaches to financing its costs. At first, existing life insurance companies took on some of the task and developed health insurance divisions within their organizations. Beginning with the New Deal in the 1930s, there was strong advocacy for nationalizing health insurance. Physicians, however, were adamantly opposed to a program controlled by the government. They proffered a corporate insurance model instead.

The life insurance companies, securely ensconced in American life, did not wish to engage in this contentious public battle between doctors and government, although they also opposed a national system. Health insurers broke off and formed their own industry. As described by Chapin, the central policies of the physicians and insurance companies were threefold:

- "Physicians . . . were financially rewarded for providing as many services as possible . . . insurers lacked authority to even question, much less regulate, physician practices."[81]
- "Fragmented care emerged . . . Insurers were prohibited from contracting with multi-specialty organizations . . . Today, if a physician encounters difficulty with a chronically ill patient or tricky-to-diagnose individual, the simplest course of action is to refer the patient to another doctor or specialist. If the patient never receives adequate care or a proper diagnosis, no one practitioner is responsible for or would likely even know the patient's final health outcome."[82]
- "Insurance companies forged overlapping institutions with doctors and hospitals . . . insurance companies gradually assumed the role of managers attempting to supervise the work of employees, in this case, physicians and hospital administrators."[83]

Employers and unions in the United States began to offer insurance benefits to their respective employees and members, assuring loyalty. The corporatized system controlled by physicians, hospitals, employers, unions, and insurers fought off even modest reforms and government interference until 1965. The late Harvard Business School professor Clayton Christensen explained that, rather than providing continuity by integrating interventions, this system "pits independent caregivers into a zero-sum, I-win-only-if-you-lose game."[84]

In this atmosphere, the national health insurance approach lost out. In 1965, however, the insufficient number of older adults covered by private insurance led to the passage of Medicare. Policymakers recognized that it would be impossible to get a national healthcare plan passed and that they should avoid the additional political issue of governmental control over its administration, so they turned to existing health insurers to administer the program on its behalf. As Chapin wrote, "although insurers initially operated in the healthcare field entirely dependent on the goodwill and support of doctors and hospital leaders, they gradually converted that relationship to obtain authority over service providers."[85]

In 1986, in response to the rise of managed care plans in the private sector, a new option, the Medicare Advantage Plan (formally, Part C), was added to basic Medicare. As McGuire et al.[86] noted, this gave "beneficiaries a choice of health insurance plans beyond the fee-for-service Medicare program." Medicare Advantage Plans are risk-based private insurance plans that take full responsibility for their enrollees' care on a prospective basis. They set up networks of participating providers and often offer additional services, such as eyeglasses. Recognizing that social context and services are critical determinants of care, some large Medicare Advantage Plans have partnered with affordable housing[87] as well as food banks and organizations offering dental services, vision screenings, and immunizations. While their efforts have been piecemeal and based on Industrial Age models, they seem to move toward the kind of broad interventions that a company like DAC will provide.

Even as healthcare moves into its digital phase, it is difficult to imagine that government, through some kind of nationalized system, will finally take over full responsibility because private health insurers are so deeply embedded in our present approach. It is quite likely that health insurers themselves will evolve from their current focus on controlling acute care to greater coverage of chronic conditions through digitization. A model such as DAC is an opportunity to integrate the components of what has become an adversarial relationship between providers and insurers. Risk, funding, service provision, and community engagement will have the opportunity to come together—by joint ventures, mergers, acquisitions, or fraught battles. For the first time in the United States, the Industrial Age segregation of intrinsically related areas of health and aging care will dissolve, and the components will come together.

Hospitals

The number of hospitals is diminishing. In 1975, there were about 1.5 million hospital beds in the United States. As of this writing, there are about 920,000.[88] Even more telling is that in 2018, as compared to the 1960s, there were about one-quarter the number of U.S. hospital beds per 1,000 people.[89] As they diminish in number, and as stays are shorter, hospitals no longer play the central role in community health that they did in the 20th century. The demise of hospitals correlates with the fading of their original purpose of battling acute disease. While the traditional hospital paradigm enabled us to conquer many terrible plagues, it is fundamentally inadequate for today and tomorrow. The societal dynamics within which the hospitals were originally built has also changed. Industrialization and other factors have led to a demographic flow to urban centers, decreasing the population served by rural hospitals.

As described in Chapter 11, the hospital acute care framework developed in the Industrial Age came to be at cross-purposes with the needs of older adults in the Era of Extended Chronic Conditions. Specialization, particularly in procedures in large city hospitals, rose to incredible levels. In 1989, to help control hospital inpatient Medicare costs, a new reimbursement scheme was implemented based on the principal diagnosis for the client's admission. It provided a fixed dollar amount to the hospital based on the number of days it would take to care for the client. If the hospital discharged a person earlier, it kept a surplus, although rules were added to penalize hospitals if they discharged the client too early.

Years ago, production staff on a television show called *Candid Camera* set up a meter on a table at a diner. A customer came in and ordered a cheeseburger and fries. The waitress said, "You can pay the set price or you can pay based on the time recorded on the meter." The customer chose the meter, which had been set to tick loudly at a very fast pace. Actors sat on either side of the customer, asking him to pass the ketchup or the salt, constantly interrupting his gobbling down his food. The customer started stuffing his mouth as quickly as possible, increasingly more frustrated and giving the audience a good laugh.

In the less comic world of healthcare, the eagerness of providers to speed up admissions and discharges became dizzying to customers. The multiple comorbidities of many frail clients, leading to longer stays than expected, also became more frustrating to the institutions. Hospitals became ever more selective about who could be admitted and for how long. Because adapting existing hospital infrastructures is often impractical and too expensive, hospitals that were overly specialized or designed around large volumes of set routines were often abandoned.

People may presume, accustomed as they are to the dominance of the Industrial Age hospital, that hospitals will incorporate lower levels of care into their systems to bolster their finances and fill their empty beds. However, this is not a likely outcome. First, many of the existing deliverers of care have become so specialized that they no longer touch or overlap sufficiently to allow for combinations or shared services. The belief that the hospital's operating systems will integrate less remunerative kinds of care also ignores the high costs of running a hospital. Hospitals do occasionally attempt to offer lower levels of care, such as operating a nursing home in order to speed the discharge of patients after surgery and perhaps to capture the nursing home rehabilitation revenue. Yet, their programs often cannot compete with outside providers whose different operating systems enable them to provide the same options at less cost. The hospitals' less-intense offerings tend to wither, and the external options grow.

It is not as if we no longer need hospitals. Acute and infectious conditions have not disappeared. We will always need the incredible sophistication of modern acute care. Chronic care often includes acute care episodes. Even with increasingly sophisticated ongoing interventions, it will not be possible to avoid all crises in people with diminished reserves. The race is on now to decentralize healthcare's sophisticated structures and skilled personnel in order to reach disparate, dispersed populations. The future is in flexibility, monitoring, and providing resources in time to resolve challenges. Some larger city systems will extend their acute care services to distant regions through efficient transportation of patients and specialists, telemedicine, and the establishment of smaller-scale local venues for acute care. Rather than concentrated bastions, the built environment will consist of distributed nodes in neural networks. Technology and skilled personnel will spread through the community.

Some hospitals are already utilizing outpatient clinical centers. One afternoon in 2021, my wife of 50 years received a FaceTime call from our son. Excited to share the call with me in an adjacent room, she jumped up quickly, took a step or two, fainted, and swan-dived onto her nose. (I later told my son to please stop calling his mother.) Her glasses cut her nose, and we did not know why she had lost

consciousness. We called her doctor, who told us to go to the local urgent care office a few blocks away. We were met by a nurse, an x-ray
technician, and a physician who did a workup.

Waiting for the roving plastic surgeon to arrive to put some
stitches in her nose, we had some time to talk to the urgent care physician. He had been an emergency department doctor for decades at
major regional hospitals, until the pressure and frustrations became
too burdensome. A hedge fund had purchased more than 20 urgent
care centers and was building more. He signed on to manage our
local unit for a piece of the financial return that the hedge fund was
expecting.

The plastic surgeon arrived. (He was also an expert in hair replacement surgery, and I didn't like the way he looked at my shining
forehead.) After the stitching, we were sent to the emergency department of a large hospital, with more extensive equipment, to be
checked out further for underlying causes of the fainting.

In the hospital, my wife was placed in an emergency area bed
and hooked up to monitors and an IV. She was never officially admitted to the hospital as a patient. It became clear that because she had
lost some weight and added more exercise to her daily routine, her
blood pressure medication dosage was too high, which caused the
fainting. (My suggestion was for her to gain weight and stop exercis-
ing.) Her own doctor discontinued her blood pressure medication the
following week.

The urgent care facility had assumed many responsibilities that
would previously have been done at the hospital. For many clients,
the urgent care would have been sufficient. I assume that in a few
years the equipment now available exclusively at the hospital will be
available at the local office, and there will be no hospital visit at all
for such an occurrence.

Increasingly, patients are no longer congregated in the 20th-cen-
tury acute care system's heavily siloed hospitals, but remain in their
communities, serviced by a newly evolving delivery system. The new
kind of digital operating system I am advocating will collect and analyze large amounts of overlapping interrelated data from physical
venues distributed throughout the community. The system will be
population based, meaning that its financial responsibilities will not
be contained within the walls of an edifice but will extend out to

thousands residing in the community. It will have financial and philosophical incentives to keep people in their homes in the community safely, less expensively, and for the long term.

The hope is that networks will increasingly connect a person's ongoing status with acute care settings. Many of the roles formerly provided by hospitals will cease, allowing surviving hospitals to become more efficient in the services that remain appropriate, and communities will continue to invest in the centers that extend those services to wider geographic catchment areas.

Hospice and Palliative Care

Hospice and palliative care are telling examples of attempts to create care for chronic conditions in the context of our acute care system. The concept of hospice as a system to help the incurably ill has been evolving since the 11th century.* In the 1950s, London-based Dame Cicely Saunders' vision, according to Nicole F. Roberts, was to address the "specific mental, physical and emotional needs. . . . by removing people with terminal diagnoses from the sterile hospital environments . . . to their home with loved ones."[90]

Hospice came to the United States with Elisabeth Kübler-Ross's groundbreaking 1969 bestseller, *On Death and Dying*. A native of Switzerland, where people died more comfortably at home, her advocacy

> . . . overturned how physicians treat dying patients . . . death was a taboo subject and discussing it was considered morbid. Patients died alone in hospitals; physicians ignored them; and adequate pain medication was underused. The book . . . pressed for more humane treatment of the dying . . . rocked the medical profession—and at the same time also resulted in a public outcry for compassionate care of the dying.[91]

In 1983, the Medicare hospice benefit was signed into law and later became a nationally guaranteed benefit for people who receive

---

*The word "hospice" derives from Latin *hospitum*, meaning hospitality or place of rest and protection for the ill and weary. Historians believe the first hospices originated in Malta around 1065 and were dedicated to caring for the ill and dying en route to and from the Holy Land. ("Hospice." Wikipedia. https://en.wikipedia.org/wiki/Hospice.)

Medicare and are terminally ill. The official government booklet states that in hospice "a specially trained team of professionals and caregivers provide care for the 'whole person,' including physical, emotional, social, and spiritual needs . . . Services typically include physical care, counseling, drugs, equipment, and supplies for the terminal illness and related conditions."[92]

Focused on the last months of life, hospice care has been a major example of utilizing the Law of Interchangeable Interventions. Hospice provides comprehensive comfort care as well as family support for a person with a terminal illness whose doctor believes he or she has a short time to live. In hospice, attempts to cure the person's illness are stopped. The turn to *caring* as opposed to *curing*—with social interventions supplementing, if not replacing, medical ones—has been well received.

The field of palliative care grew out the hospice movement, utilizing the same principles of improving the quality of life of patients and their families by relieving the pain, symptoms, and stress of a serious or debilitating illness. So far, the Medicare hospice benefit has been offered only to individuals on Medicare diagnosed with a terminal illness who agree to forgo further "curative" treatments. Some health insurers provide various types of palliative services to participants who do not qualify for hospice. With palliative care, as opposed to hospice, a person does not have to give up treatment that might cure a serious illness. It can be provided along with curative treatment and may begin at the time of diagnosis. Often insurers cover only some services such as pain management but do not provide for home visits, coordination of care, or social and spiritual counseling. This inconsistency seems to come from concerns about introducing coverage for chronic care into an acute care system. While it may often be the case that palliative care would reduce the costs of medical interventions, it does so by opening the back door to nonmedical, perhaps even social, interventions. Providers are concerned about potential precedents that will lead to greater expenses.

Although many practitioners working with chronically ill patients utilize palliative care approaches, confusion is caused by a common misunderstanding that one needs to be "terminal" to receive palliative care. Both inadequate insurance coverage and insufficient numbers of professionals trained in palliative care prevent such services to be rendered to a large portion of the individuals living with chronic and advanced disease who could have their quality (and quantity) of life improved, frequently at dramatically reduced costs. Although there is no organized political opposition to the use of palliative care, its slow, truncated adoption is a product of our history. The necessary community participation and resources must be developed.

Looking back, hospice was an early exception in allowing non-medical, and even social, interventions to be reimbursed during an acute care–focused era. Palliative care extended the same kind of services, even if people were not terminally ill. It is inevitable that palliative care and hospice will be integrated more fully in community-based network systems of care. They may be subcontracted to separate agencies, or the care network itself may bring the services in-house, as is the case with the PACE program, discussed in Chapter 7. As community care for chronic conditions incorporates greater ranges of interventions, the former islands of hospice and palliation will be integrated as standard options.

Government

Not only are insurers and providers turning to address the new realities, so are governmental policymakers. The tragic consequences of COVID-19 in nursing homes and assisted living facilities laid bare the undeniable fact that such institutions are not always safe havens for older adults. By early 2022, "over 200,000 residents and staff in long-term care facilities [had] died from COVID-19."[93] People with comorbidities living in compressed physical proximity and cared for by underpaid caregivers rendered the older residents sitting ducks for contagion. The COVID-19 pandemic is another factor that shows us that the time has come to create a new arena for aging in the United States.

It has become clear to government that despite the heroics of U.S. hospitals in addressing the crisis of the pandemic, both the problem of contagion and its solution lie in the community. For a long while, masks and social distancing were the basic tools to contain or slow the spread of the disease. The lack of compliance with these simple requirements laid bare our lack of community networking. Despite the insufficient number of hospital beds during the periods of highest infection rates in various communities, the solution is not to create more hospital beds, but rather to develop medical resources within underlying communities that will keep people from needing hospitals. The next battles will be fought not within our medical industrial complexes but among the civilian population. It will be a guerrilla campaign, winning the hearts and minds of the people and marshaling the resources within communities to respond to the new threats.

Realizing our vulnerability to COVID-19, the government began tracking and orchestrating the supply chains necessary to produce vaccines and personal protective equipment for health workers and the community. Many people recovering in the hospital needed to be discharged to free up beds but were still not ready to return back to the community. New centers were established to coordinate the wait for their safe return. The distribution of the vaccine to hundreds of millions presented problems of how to coordinate delivery, how to reach inaccessible and resistant populations, and how to develop communication and continuity. The best responses involved developing networks of information. The U.S. Department of Health and Human Services set up a volunteer Medical Reserve Corps (https:// aspr.hhs.gov/MRC/Pages/index.aspx), for example, for retired and underutilized medical personnel, somewhat like the National Guard, to be trained and at the ready for emergencies. Such networks will spill over and will come to predominate aging care in our communities. I picture a future in which existing government healthcare bureaucracies, like the oppressive draft boards of the 1960s, will transform into something we haven't yet fully imagined.

Nursing Homes

As described above in this chapter, nursing homes have also become more medicalized, following changes in government reimbursement patterns. Stays in nursing homes are shorter because people do not enter until they are already very frail and sick. As states reduce Medicaid reimbursements for long-term care, community-based nonprofit nursing homes—in order to survive—are becoming institutions for short-term rehabilitation or end-of-life care. Government financing is accelerating this change.

As nursing homes turned more to Medicare, the reimbursement system was changed to become more aligned with the payment system of hospitals. Previously, Medicare reimbursement for rehabilitation in nursing homes was based on the number of direct therapy minutes. In 2020, the government implemented a new system, PDPM (Patient Driven Payment Model), assigning a classification to each resident based on a projected number of days of care rather than therapy minutes.[94] The home is incentivized to control costs because if it takes shorter or longer periods to obtain a desired result, the home experiences a surplus or loss accordingly. Even for the Medicaid patient, in order to keep afloat financially, the Resource Utilization Group (RUG) system described in Chapter 7 forces the home to give preference to people who have more complex and expensive needs, for which the home will receive higher compensation, rather than allowing the Law of Interchangeable Interventions to access less costly and less medical choices that are more beneficial to the residents.

The increasing number of frail older adults creates pressure on government resources. In response, the administrative arms of government continue to tighten regulatory requirements and shrink reimbursements. The range of each level of care in nursing homes is becoming narrower, with greater financial risk when not enough clients fit the more frail profiles. A specialized level is less able to address clients' more comprehensive needs. This change in institutional function is distancing nonprofit nursing homes from their underlying communities, who have been using them as the residences of their older relatives rather than places for short stays. The homes are then less able to raise capital from their local communities, who no longer have the same sense of connection and loyalty.

As these developments continue, hedge funds and proprietary chains will purchase nursing homes and assisted living facilities, focus on short-term Medicare services, and reduce operating costs by standardizing operations. The chronic custodial care traditionally offered by nonprofit homes will decrease, as we have already seen. Ironically, despite the fact that this is an era of chronic care, nursing homes are less appropriate or available to offer traditional long-term care and have become more focused on acute care.

In addition to the problems of specialization and cost, the COVID-19 experience has brought national attention to some of the serious drawbacks of the traditional nursing home setting, as well as the governmental attention mentioned in the previous section. With shared bedrooms and crowded spaces, the density of interaction among residents with multiple chronic conditions and weaker defenses against infection turned many nursing homes into death pits.[95] The marketing of nursing home beds and the staffing shortages have become even more difficult, including, as Gleckman described, "the inability of family members to visit clients during a lock-down . . . and high costs at a time of widespread infection."[96] Residents are increasingly isolated in their rooms to minimize infection, making the experience even more depressing than it already has been. Increased expenses also occur from the need to redesign spaces for infection control and to increase wages in order to attract labor into these dangerous environments. It is particularly tragic that an infectious disease ravages facilities for chronic conditions in an era dominated by chronic conditions. This sudden shocking event will set the stage for a shift in public expectations of nursing homes as central repositories of frail older people.

In the future, as nursing homes become a less appropriate and available option, enterprises like DAC will assume responsibility for deploying the Medicare and Medicaid payments available for frail older adults. Nursing homes will have to compete with other, less expensive noninstitutional settings for rehabilitation services, for example. Eventually, there will be dramatically fewer nursing home beds for the older person who simply needs shelter and food and a little looking after, but whose condition does not provide adequate government reimbursement for the expenses of a nursing home. Presently, that person must find those needs addressed elsewhere. Companies like DAC will step into the breach to help many of them meet those needs while staying in the community, an alternative that the older adult prefers anyway, and that will save us all a lot of money.

Rivington House

Rivington House in New York provides an example of how the Law of Interchangeable Interventions sometimes plays out unseen. Public School 20 opened in 1899, in the Lower East Side neighborhood of Manhattan, to serve poor immigrant children living nearby in crowded and decaying tenements. The building was made of brick and terra-cotta in a style designed to bring in more air and light. In 1995, Villagecare, a nonprofit nursing home operator, accessed a $70 million state-backed bond to convert the building from a school to an HIV/AIDS nursing home, calling it Rivington House.

In 2015, Villagecare sold the building to the Allure Group, a proprietary enterprise, for $28 million, absorbing $17.7 of Villagecare's debts. Allure paid the city another $16 million to remove a deed restriction that had limited the building to use as a nonprofit residential healthcare facility. Allure then sold the building for $118 million to a luxury developer who planned to create about 100 luxury apartments.[97]

There was a great public consternation when the deed restriction was removed. Looking beyond the public outrage, the legal wrangling, and the political ramifications, one sees the Law of Interchangeable Interventions at work. The building had been built, renovated, and adapted to address a succession of different needs: first as a school; then as a Medicaid nursing home serving the HIV/AIDS community; and when Medicaid rates were no longer adequate for organizational survival, as an HIV/AIDS hospice. When the discovery of drug cocktails arose as an intervention that enabled people with HIV/AIDS to remain in the community, the hospice was no longer needed.

The $70 million state investment for the 1985 conversion to a nursing home had been made under the assumption that nursing homes would be needed forever. There was little societal comprehension then of the march of new interventions or the coming medicalization of long-term care. Yet, as the reimbursement system changed and traditional nursing homes became ever more specialized, and as new options were introduced into the care of HIV/AIDS clients, there were insufficient revenues to keep Villagecare's operation financially above water. The Law of Interchangeable Interventions determined that better alternatives were available for the former residents of the building.

Society at large does not see or understand this broad shift, however. The technical adjustments to reimbursements have set in motion a chain of results for which the cause-and-effect sequence is not immediately visible. No one, including those responsible for the reimbursement changes, comprehended the impact of the state's new policy on the long-term care industry. The other bureaus of government also did not realize that, after a century of governmental investment in and *partnership with community facilities owned by nonprofit community organizations, the state had effectively abandoned nursing homes, making it necessary to find different interventions for their clients. Government stopped paying for capital improvements and—rather than continuing to view this archipelago of community organizations as partners—stripped out reimbursements, swapping their established commitments for a focus on reducing government's annual operational costs. The closing of Rivington House removed those beds from the Medicaid rolls and saved approximately $18 million per year in Medicaid costs.*

Government was responding to rising financial obligations resulting from demographic changes. It was also responding to the reality that underlying communities were changing as well. As the World War II generation of builders and investors in community institutions died out, their children and grandchildren moved away from their neighborhoods. Community organizations no longer had the ability to make the necessary ongoing capital investments. Nor did these community organizations retain well-placed community advocates to influence government officials. They were no longer appropriate partners to government.

The Disappearance of Community Involvement in American Aging

In the early years of Medicaid, from 1965 and even into the 1980s, nursing homes tended to emanate from and be controlled by their local communities. Upstanding middle-class families would feel ashamed if they placed Mom on Medicaid in a nursing home. By 1985 or so, the ethic had reversed. A middle-class family was viewed as foolish if they did not avail themselves of vehicles to set aside and retain Mom's assets in order to access Medicaid. Elder law attorneys in the community who counseled families on how to maintain Mom's assets became valued fiduciaries similar to investment advisors. While the nursing home continued to hold out that it was a community asset, families learned to see it as a public utility, expecting that their prior group identification and engagement would secure access to the facility.

But as Medicaid reimbursement levels continued to fall below the actual cost of care, new sources of income were sought. Nursing homes reached beyond their traditional lower-income constituencies to find more lucrative private payers. Community leadership shifted its focus from raising community funds to hiring consultants who could help secure better governmental reimbursement. As the middle class increasingly moved to the suburbs, communities no longer felt sufficient engagement with new facilities to attract charitable donations. For-profit chains rose to avail themselves of the opportunity to fill some of the new void. Community involvement dissipated and government was left with virtually sole responsibility for American aging.

Perhaps what is most curious is the nature of the public outcry over the sale of the Rivington House building. Even if nothing that occurred was illegal, the windfall profits and the inaccurate, self-serving statements made by Allure were enraging. Community leaders felt betrayed and wished to reverse the transaction and return the building to an earlier function for which there was actually no longer sufficient demand, or to demand future investment for something they could not even define. Their pronouncements reflected a lack of understanding of the ongoing dynamic at play in the world of aging. Melissa Aase, executive director of the University Settlement, an organization providing social services to low-income families, older adults, and youth, stated, "We're going to keep trying to fight for the building to come back to the community." Manhattan Borough President Gale Brewer noted, "the Rivington House's value to the community far exceeded $16 million . . . and there is much work to be done to create needed nursing home beds in the community."[98]

The public was shocked by the loss of a building that to them represented community commitment to frail older neighbors. They did not realize that its use as a nursing home had already become outdated. The building was no longer tenable as a Medicaid nursing home. In fact, changing governmental reimbursements had forced the facility to reach out to a much wider geographic area and to garner more acutely ill clients, so Rivington House no longer served only clients and families who lived nearby. It had lost its direct and immediate ties to its former local community. With the gentrification of the neighborhood, as evidenced by the demand that Allure recognized for an upscale housing development, Rivington House also lost its tie to the local labor market. In effect, it was no longer a community facility, even before Allure arrived. The public outcry led to the abandonment of the planned conversion to luxury condos. Eventually, the New York State Public Health and Health Planning Council approved the transformation of Rivington House to a psychiatric and drug abuse program under the umbrella of a major hospital, but even this was not satisfactory to the community. Neighbors to Save Rivington House, a local community group, stated "if (the proposed new plan) does not include nursing home (sic) it will not meet this neighborhood's need . . . for all or a portion of the building to be returned to the community for use for nursing home beds . . ."[99]

Rivington House is a revealing story of the Law of Interchangeable Interventions in action. Originally created as a local long-term care facility, a constant drumbeat of new, less expensive interventions continually pushed out what was being provided. The facility survived by constantly moving to more expensive, more medicalized uses, eventually becoming part of a hospital. In the end, it could not continue. The societal changes that underlay the evolution remained unrecognized by the different arms of the government, by the organizational leadership, and by the community. That is the underlying pathos of the story.

Without a deep understanding of the nature of the aging dynamic, we lose the opportunity to develop overall strategies that allow us to capture and redeploy assets, and we become victims to short-term tactical moves. Because the present situation of aging is not clear to most of us, we fumble forward blindly, angered by the loss of the old and not realizing that it no longer operates as we believe it does. When we have a clear perception of how aging is changing, we will be better able to convert existing resources.

Assisted Living

As nursing homes have fewer places for long-term clients, some higher-functioning older adults move into assisted living. A region's assisted living facilities most often come under the control of a few, very efficient corporate operators who replicate the exact same operating procedures throughout all their facilities. Within them, the same dynamic will unfold as in nursing homes. As the assisted living facilities serve a population that is too healthy for nursing homes but less healthy than the previous assisted living cadre, these homes will become more medicalized, more expensive, and eventually more exclusive. Fewer people will be appropriate candidates for residence. Many clients who would formerly have settled in assisted living will stay in their communities and seek out more interventions at home. DAC will be right there to help them.

Continuing Care Retirement Communities

In the mid-20th century, some religious and other nonprofit associations developed a model for old-age housing and care called the Continuing Care Retirement Community (CCRC). These were campuses primarily for wealthy older clients who paid a large fee (hundreds of thousands of dollars) to buy into the community, followed by substantial monthly charges, for the use of an independent living townhouse or apartment for the remainder of their lives. With this came a guarantee that the monthly charge would not change if and when the resident needed care in the community's assisted living or nursing home. Upon a resident's death, CCRCs refunded to the estate all or part of the original buy-in fee. This arrangement combined housing, some healthcare, and nursing home insurance. Governments tended to like the CCRC model because of the built-in private nursing home coverage. Thousands of CCRC campuses were built.

As the strength, sophistication, and reach of the new digital aging network grows, the demand for gated CCRCs will diminish. People wealthy enough to buy into a CCRC will have the alternative of purchasing different levels of coverage from the aging care network while continuing to live at home, rather than moving to a CCRC. They will have the same kind of guaranteed rate from a company like DAC, no matter how much care they need. The CCRCs' assurances of future nursing home access will become less prized, as short-term rehabilitation services and other interventions will be readily available and life at home can be made satisfactory. The CCRC's three-level structure of care, including independent living, assisted living, and nursing home, will lose its relevance as the digitized aging network can drop in and manage wider ranges of tailored services in other environments. Many families of CCRC residents also have ended up paying additional costs for support services to keep family members out of the CCRC nursing home. Now, the aging network will pick that up. The CCRC's ability to create and sustain social connections will no longer be an exclusive advantage, as people continue to live in their old neighborhoods, within their long-term social groups, now bolstered by the connective tissue of DAC.

Some CCRCs will respond to changing circumstances by contracting with the new aging networks. A few will continue to thrive because they have created strong social connections. Many others, however, are likely to lose their ability to fill vacancies as residents die off, and they will have to close their doors.

Homecare

Until now, homecare, which has included everything from assistance with activities of daily living to nursing care and physical therapy, has generally been provided by private agencies. Their business covers a great variety of clients in different work conditions and locations, and their labor force does difficult work for fairly low pay. Homecare aides need to be reliable and competent and to treat clients with compassion and humor. If an older adult hires a homecare aide who helps him or her out of bed and assists with intimate activities, his or her life will be much better if that person is someone the client likes. And if the older person's life is better, his or her spirits are likely to be higher, and the person is probably healthier. Each client has so many variables in health needs and personality preferences that the typical homecare agency has not been able to manage more than a few hundred clients at a time. A newer business model, however, could accumulate a larger database of caregivers to match with a larger number of clients and develop programs that would quickly suggest lists of appropriate matches.

In the traditional agency model, the agency interviews a prospective client and assesses the home situation and the family's resources. Then, the aide who seems to be the best fit, based on anecdotal evidence and personal experience, is sent into the home. In a digital platform model, an agent will do an assessment in the same fashion but can also feed information into a large database that compares the client with others who have the same conditions and preferences. The client's profile can be matched with caregivers who have worked successfully with older adults whose profiles are similar. Using a digital program that can compare thousands of previous matches will pinpoint a much more finely tuned group of choices, rather than depending solely on the agency's intuition. Putting the client's data together with the homecare professionals' information will result in a digital matching service that combines the best attributes of a ridesharing company and a dating app.

While previously it was almost impossible to supervise the decentralized work of aides going into homes, there can now be ongoing feedback and analysis in real time using various devices. Visits and procedures can be tracked, complaints and compliments registered, creating a robust network of ongoing information and support for both client and caregiver.

Using digital tools to map an older adult's needs in the course of the day can fine-tune the fit between clients and homecare professionals. Maybe it's best for a particular client to have a team of aides, each of whom performs a different function at the time of the day when it is needed. This reduces the number of hours that aides spend with an individual and allows someone who is an expert at administering meds, giving massages, or reading aloud to plan an efficient schedule for delivering their expertise to multiple clients. Homecare nurses, for example, will have apps that can lay out the logistics of the day: the route, estimated times of arrival, expected times for administering interventions, and completed tasks. Everyone on the nurse's route will be notified of expected arrival times, changes, or delays. The efficiencies in such systems are attractive to providers as well as clients, so they will undoubtedly be developed very soon, much as they are already in place for package delivery and ride sharing.

The frustrations of homecare work as presently configured and its low wages exacerbate the homecare labor shortage caused by our demographics. Using a program that matches homecare workers' skills to older adults' needs more exactly will have an enormous impact on the entire aging care workforce. There are a wide range of interventions a homecare professional may perform, such as bathing, lifting, transporting, incontinence care, and dementia management, as well as housework tasks such as cleaning, laundry, and cooking. Each caregiver's inventory of skills can be matched specifically to a client's needs in a way that has not existed before. If various homecare interventions have different hourly rates, the program can quickly scan recent transactions and determine a pay rate for a particular arrangement.

One of the anachronisms of the traditional model of homecare has been that all workers in a single category have been treated as equals in terms of salary and benefits. This doesn't incentivize workers to improve skillsets. Now, homecare professionals can increase their hourly pay rate if they increase their skills. It will also be possible for them to choose their hours and duties. The new incentives will ameliorate the national shortage of caregivers. According to *Home Healthcare News*, "The number of new job openings for home health aides by 2025 is expected to reach 423,200, a growth rate of 32%." That, combined with the existing shortage, will result in a national shortage of 446,300 homecare aides by 2025.[100] With electronic processing of homecare, professionals will have more information and control of their time and tasks, with fewer surprises and frustrations. Many more individuals may come to the fore to offer their services. Millions of work hours could be added by making pay and responsibilities attractive to those who have been unable or unwilling to work in traditional healthcare. People who want to cook or be companions but are not skilled in physical care or nursing can supplement their incomes and serve an older adult's part-time care needs. Even neighbors could enter the system, registering the services they would like to provide and offering a foundation for informal cooperatives.

Immediate feedback on the homecare professional's performance can also be tied to his or her pay level. Just as Uber drivers and their customers can rate one another, so can homecare professionals and their clients. It may be that a homecare professional with a higher rating can bid more successfully for clients and for more pay. Conversely, families rated as more reasonable and appreciative will attract higher-rated homecare professionals.

Collecting large amounts of data can reveal patterns that are not immediately obvious. Electronic data might indicate to a homecare operator, for example, that demand for aides shoots up on weekends but their availability falls off, despite the fact that a higher rate of pay is offered. The managers may at first assume the lack of available aides is caused by homecare professionals wanting to spend weekends with their families. But when additional questions are programmed in, it turns out that weekends are the time when many difficult family members visit the clients, creating stressful interactions. The data can sometimes reveal what individual managers cannot see.

The information database and the possibility of tracking the workday will ease the anxiety that stems from the idea of an unsupervised stranger in the home of a vulnerable older person. Accurate and ongoing feedback to all relevant parties will be a great source of comfort.

Conclusion

Having reviewed the range of healthcare options for older adults, it is clear that collecting large amounts of data will be necessary for all of them. This will require a dramatic restructuring of the training and educational systems for health professionals, tailored to a dramatically different human care–delivery system. Training and educational programs for healthcare professionals in the United States were designed to meet the needs of the previous Industrial Age acute care–delivery system. As a consequence, the various disciplines were sequestered from one another, with sharp boundaries.

The new Digital Age chronic care–delivery system will require professionals who, while grounded in their particular disciplines, are also cross-trained to understand and communicate with others. All will require a new global vision of the future of care delivery in the United States, oriented to the transmigrations of populations and the variety of interventions among and between traditional disciplines and venues. Care will be shaped by multidisciplinary teams cross-trained to understand the range of possible interventions. Historic professional attributes based on rigidity and boundary protection will give way to attributes such as the ability to adapt to new techniques and roles; the skill to coordinate with other professional disciplines; and comfort in translating information to older adults, families, and communities with whom they maintain trusting relationships.

The new networked aging system will shorten and tighten feedback loops. It will integrate consumers, providers, payers, and regulators, who will see the results of initiatives quickly and be able to adapt. This will not occur neatly. There will be unanticipated gaps, problems, and sometimes unexpected negative consequences. There will be calls to return to the tried-and-true methods. There will be reversals and loss of nerve, but the old frameworks will inexorably give way as new ones emerge.

CHAPTER 14

Government Aging Policy

If a government policy is not just a set of legislative enactments, administrative interpretations, and judicial rulings but is more the way that these various and sundry determinations come to shape our actual experience, then United States policy for aging care is no longer appropriate and must be dramatically reformulated. In 1965, Congress responded to the outcry for a national response to the needs of its older adults by instituting Medicare and Medicaid. For some, a fervent desire burns for a repeat of that kind of national "Big Bang" in order to reset the way we care for our oldest generation. Such an eventuality is unlikely, however. Medicare and Medicaid were passed at a unique moment in American life when there was an ascendant economy on the world stage, the enormous Baby Boomer generation was coming to adulthood, and one party controlled all three branches of the federal government. No one yet suspected what the future demographic and economic significance of the older population would bring.

Even if such a monumental reset were to occur again, it would soon be bereft of efficacy. In the political environment of the early 2020s, the minority political party, in order to deny the majority any success, thwarts all revisions and refinements necessary to implement and refine an expansive new program. Even if a new system is somehow enacted into law, it will surely be on the opposition's hit list and so not result in the kind of long-term systemic change that was accomplished by the original Medicare and Medicaid legislation.

Pressure from the new size and needs of the aging population is arising from a number of directional forces. Given their immensity and complexity, it is possible only to speculate on exactly how they will shape governmental postures. But while specific government responses are currently unknowable, it is highly likely that they will be directed by demographic, financial, technical, and sociological developments. Government will no longer be aging's primary driver, but it will assume the role of attempting to protect consumers by reining in and redirecting egregious practices in the system of caring for older people. Some of the most important areas in which federal and state governments will play a role are discussed in the sections that follow.

Financial Burdens on Programs and Providers

As emphasized throughout this volume, the United States is facing enormous demographic challenges from the coming numbers of older adults. Historic governmental aging policies cannot withstand the increasing weight of these demographics. The already enormous expenditures for the oldest cohort of the population (see Chapter 6) hide the unsustainability of the current programs. The Social Security Trust Fund is projected to be depleted in 2034.[101] Because of increased longevity, the contributions of Boomers to the fund during their working years have been inadequate to cover the full length of their retirement years. The year 2022 was the first time the benefits paid out were larger than the contributions deposited into the Trust. It is estimated that if the program remains the same, benefits will come solely from payroll taxes on the decreasing ratio of workers to retirees (see the aging pyramids in Chapter 1). As a result, in 2034, benefits will be reduced to an estimated 78% of current levels (adjusted for inflation).

The negative impact of such a reduction would be profound for millions of older Americans. In 2021, "37 percent of men and 42 percent of women on Social Security . . . (got) 50 percent or more of their income from the program."[102] In order to maintain full benefits beyond 2034, Congress has a number of possible options to consider, such as raising taxes on various constituencies or increasing retirement age. Each of those approaches carries differential burdens on various groups, so the debate will be hotly contentious.

Social Security is highly popular, but given the stasis in Congress at the time of this writing it is not at all clear when or if adjustments will be made to maintain its full benefits in the future. After all, when passed, Social Security benefits were said to be one leg of a three-legged stool consisting of Social Security, private pensions, and savings. This is no longer true, given that private sources have been drastically reduced. Nevertheless, a residual historical belief remains in some parts of the American body politic that if one of those legs becomes shorter it is the sole responsibility of the individual to make up for it, whatever the underlying causation or economic realities.[103]

Medicare, the foundational program for medical care and hospitalization for older adults, will experience financial disruption even earlier than Social Security, in 2026. The annual 2021 Medicare Trustees Report included the following:

- The 2020 $495.5 billion Medicare shortfall constituted about 16% of the federal deficit.
- Medicare has a $5.95 trillion cumulative cash shortfall since 1965, which Medicare covers from other programs.
- "Medicare's cash shortfall is responsible for one-third of the federal debt."[104]

An even more immediate impact on older men and women will be the financial stress on nursing homes caused by Medicaid shortfalls. According to Spanko (2019), "Medicaid accounted for exactly two-thirds, or 67.6%, of resident days in the third quarter of 2019."[105] The program is partially financed by state governments that often face financial difficulties and, unlike the federal government, must balance their budgets. A Medicaid bed in a nursing home is the last refuge for many older adults. According to Osterland (2021), "About 70% of people over age 65 will need some form of long-term care before they die."[106] The average yearly cost of a private nursing home bed in 2021 was $107,000.[107] But according to estimates by the Government Accountability Office, "nearly half (48%) of households headed by someone 55 and older lack some form of retirement savings."[108] "Of those who have saved, roughly one-quarter have less than $100,000 in retirement accounts."[109] So they have no funds to pay for the nursing home beds they may need. Nursing homes are almost completely dependent on the funds they receive from the unreliable Medicaid and Medicare. Furthermore, in part because Boomers generally will not tolerate existing institutional environments, they have moved to the 800,000 assisted-living beds in the United States, and so nursing homes have lost many clients who were paying their own way. In assisted living facilities, the average cost was $54,000 a year in 2021.

Even though the costs are half that of nursing homes,[110] those less expensive settings are not available to perhaps 50% or more of the older population because most states do not extend Medicaid into assisted living.

Medicare pays for geriatric care so inadequately that even doctors are hard to find, as noted in Chapter 9. Geriatricians constitute only a small portion of America's 1 million physicians. As of 2021, the geriatrician workforce capacity in the United States had actually decreased from 10,270 in 2000 to 8,502 in 2010 to approximately 7,300, of whom only 50% practiced full-time. The American Geriatrics Society estimates that the United States will need 30,000 geriatricians by 2030.[111]

Marc Zimmet, president and CEO of Zimmet Healthcare Services Group, has found that nursing home providers are voluntarily taking beds off service and then reporting the reduced capacity to federal authorities. The reduced maximum capacity bed count artificially inflates the occupancy rate and, according to Zimmet, "inaccurately portrays a service sector that is smaller than it actually is,"[112] thereby downplaying the industry's actual distress and reducing the state's inclination to give relief by increasing Medicaid rates. Some estimate that average pre-pandemic occupancy rates of 80% may be as low as 50%–60% in many places.[113]

Low Medicaid reimbursement rates, coupled with the financial hardships from the COVID-19 pandemic and the lack of savings by older adults, threaten the viability of the entire nursing home sector. An American Health Care Association and National Center for Assisted Living survey found that "more than half of nursing homes are currently operating at a loss and 72% of nursing homes say they won't be able to sustain operation another year at the current pace."[114]

Ironically, just as the epidemiologic era turns to chronic care, the primary setting for the long-term care of frail adults is melting away. Some of this may be related to transitory COVID effects, or it may be that the pandemic brought public awareness to underlying inadequacies that were inevitable.

The actual impact of the blows from changes in governmental funding to nursing homes is underreported. As stated by Robert Kramer, president of the consulting firm Nexus Insights, "there never will come a time when we will return to the old normal."[115] David

Yeske, past chair of the Finance Planning Association, noted, "In this political climate, I don't see a policy response for this issue on the horizon."[116] Families will no longer have Industrial Age settings and simultaneously no appropriate chronic care system to turn to.

Reviewing the Impact of Governmental Support for Nursing Homes

Rather than suddenly seeing nursing homes as a failure, it may be worthwhile to remember their important contributions to the developmental path of chronic care in the United States. As described previously, in 1965, Medicaid created for the first time a national system of facilities that cared for frail older Americans. That gathering together of more than 1 million older adults with society's developing armamentarium of available resources eventually led to the formulation of national best practices, specializations, and new understandings of chronic care. These institutional innovations fostered greater longevity among frail residents. This policy is consistent with the long American tradition of immigrants to a new land banding together, developing the resources to survive, and enabling future generations to disperse and assimilate. It has not been my experience that the professionals in the government's health bureaucracy were ignorant or uncaring. To the contrary, as described in Chapter 5, they were often working creatively, even feverishly, within a legislative framework that was so successful early on that the numbers of older adults and available interventions simply outgrew and overwhelmed that framework.

Digital Companies and Government Regulation

As described in Chapter 12, digital companies such as the hypothetical Digital Aging Care, Inc. (DAC), have developed approaches that can be adapted to address the needs of frail older adults living in the community and replace many of the institutions that dominate policy-making today. They will have the resources to invest in technology that works across multiple providers focusing on the intersection of digital technology, health services, and workforce. An article entitled "The Rise of Big Tech May Just Be Starting" stated that "the largest companies in tech . . . now seem poised to expand their reach and influence over the rest of the economy, rather than relinquish it."[117] They are using "our screens to become the primary portal through which a handful of companies capture a slice of everything we do."[118]

Apple, for example,

> Got into [the] TV business . . . the way a lot of the tech giants do a lot of things nowadays: It spent gobs of money . . . and where money wasn't enough, it used its advantages as a tech platform to help it along . . . Apple spent a reported $6 billion on content to start Apple TV+, and it gave away a free year of the service with the sale of new Apple devices . . . Apple can continue to throw money at its TV service indefinitely; it could easily afford to never make any money from TV+ and simply run the service as a kind of brand-marketing project.[119]

It is only a matter of time until these large digital companies apply their resources to the industry of caring for the nation's older adults.

Companies like DAC will bring enormous benefits to older clients at lower cost, but they will need oversight and regulation to guarantee the safety of their clients. A digital model holds dangers that are not easy to predict. It has the potential to take the control of aging and healthcare away not only from the government, but also from communities and individuals. We risk losing some of the protections that the government has traditionally attempted to assure, such as transparency, safety, and equality for older adults. The sophisticated algorithms of DAC could contain all manner of assumptions, orientations, biases, and economic distortions that would be harmful to individuals. But just as the historic array of silos of the healthcare industry has become inadequate, so have the historic governmental policies and regulations that frame and support them. It will be the role of the government to create a new framework, probably a very different one, for the new networked systems of aging care.

Governmental approaches to regulating the commercial world in the United States were originally designed to control the excesses of Gilded Age technology that arose from the development of internal combustion and the electrification of the country in the late 19th and early 20th centuries. The rules evolved through shifting judicial interpretations to address changes in modern society. The Sherman and Clayton Antitrust Acts were passed near the beginning of the 20th century to prevent large companies from restraining trade through unchecked consolidations, mergers, and other behaviors that lessened competition.* The early concerns were focused on industries such as steel, oil, and railroads. The focus was on size, and courts considered market share in forcing behemoths such as Standard Oil of New Jersey and the Hollywood studio system to divest. Certain other practices such as price-fixing and collusion were considered (and remain) illegal.

By the 1960s there was rising criticism of what was perceived to be arbitrary government antitrust enforcement. An approach developed at the University of Chicago known as the Chicago School shifted policy to maximizing consumer welfare, what Phillips Sawyer described as "the attempt to get the greatest number of goods to customers, reliably, at the lowest cost. The older concerns with safeguarding against undue political influence or preserving a high threshold of market competitors . . . largely disappeared,"[120] under the new belief that markets were self-correcting and government intervention often caused more inefficiencies rather than making them more competitive.

The Digital Age has also challenged previous approaches to antitrust regulation. Although large digital platforms have reduced the costs to consumers for a whole host of services, there is concern that the consumer-welfare standard is no longer sufficient to protect competitive and free market principles. Wheeler et al. explained:

> The "move fast and break things" mantra of Silicon Valley has meant that digital companies move fast and make their own

---

*"Technically, a trust is a legal device used to coordinate multiple property owners through a unified management structure. Business owners combine their interests into a single legal entity—the trust." (Phillips Sawyer, L. U.S. Antitrust law and policy in historical perspective. Working Paper 19-110. http://www.hbs.edu/ris/Publication%20Files/19-110_e21447ad-d98a-451f-8ef0-ba42209018e6.pdf.) Congress passed the Sherman Anti-Trust Act in 1890. This first federal law against "industrial combination and monopoly . . . began to reverse the trend toward unchecked consolidation." The legislation stated that "every contract, combination in the form of trust or otherwise, or conspiracy, in restraint of trade or commerce among the several states, or with foreign nations, is hereby declared illegal." In 1914, the Clayton Antitrust Act was passed to prohibit discrimination in prices among purchasers, exclusive deals tying a purchaser to a single supplier, and any action that "substantially lessens competition or tends to create a monopoly. At this time, the Federal Trade Commission was created to 'prevent the unlawful suppression of competition.'" (History of anti-trust regulation: Government regulation of monopolies. https://cs.stanford.edu/people/eroberts/cs181/projects/corporate-monopolies/government_history.html.)

rules. Antitrust statutes reflect a time when markets were relatively stable because technology was relatively stable. Today, the rapid pace of digital technology means companies can accumulate unbridled power and control, and can move rapidly to advantage themselves by exploiting consumers and eliminating potential competition.[121]

Nature of the New Challenge to Government Regulation

Imagine for a moment that you are the creator and czar of fractions. You invent three kinds that are altogether different: halves, thirds, and fourths. These three fractions are wonderful inventions, for they enable people to understand and piece together things that previously were left dangling, and probably had not even been visible. Imagine a time when these three fractions were supreme and absolutely inviolate. Halves would have all the ingredients of half-ness, nothing more or less. The same with thirds and quarters. The professionals in each kind of fraction live and compete only within their own entirely self-enclosed universe, preventing an understanding of the total cumulative total of all the fractions.

Then along comes the idea of a common denominator, here twelfths. Suddenly, the need to fit into halves, thirds, and fourths loses significance (although the half world still sees itself as dominant). Let's go further, to common denominators of 24ths, then 48ths, 120ths, and 120,000ths. Then someone invents a machine, let's call it a computer, that can manipulate these fractions—now called bits—and apply different combinations of them to each problem. As we look back, we realize that the halves, thirds, and fourths that so dominated us were merely convenient groupings and that the usefulness of those frameworks has passed. Of course, there remain halves, thirds, and fourths, but only rarely are they meaningful (perhaps when it is useful to gather together a variety of fractions under the old headings of half, third, or quarter). Their convenience is reduced because of the arrival of calculations, called algorithms, that manipulate those bits of information. The algorithms constantly develop more effective, less expensive combinations and so constantly change the constituent components of each of the original three fractions. New enterprises arise that break down all the elements of the universe into a common denominator, accumulate the data, and apply algorithms to a problem.

This is what has happened in chronic care. Rather suddenly hospitals, nursing homes, and homecare all become comparable and mixable in never-ending combinations to solve riddles, such as the most appropriate approach for a complex frail older adult. Their former frameworks have been superseded by algorithms that cross boundaries and change configurations of care in infinitely new ways.

As already stated, it will be the role of government to develop policies to create a new framework—probably a very different one—for the new networked systems caring for older adults. Digital networks eliminate the silos that dominated Industrial Age healthcare, and a new framework without natural or inherent curbs dominates. In *The Age of Surveillance Capitalism: The Fight for a Human Future at the New Frontier of Power*, Shoshana Zuboff described how large digital players such as Facebook and Amazon have been accumulating people's private individual experiences without proper safeguards, approval, or even recognition by customers. What she referred to as "free raw material for translation into behavioral data"[122] is an asset that is bought and sold "to nudge, coax, tune, and herd behavior toward profitable outcomes."[123] What she called surveillance capitalism gathers "vast domains of knowledge *from* us, but not *for* us."[124] It can be "a rogue force driven by novel economic imperatives that disregard social norms and nullify the elemental rights associated with individual autonomy."[125] Zuboff urged us to recognize the power of our new digital tools and to place restrictions around them in order to harness them to good purpose. She stated, "If the digital future is to be our home, then it is we who must make it so."[126]

New government policy must address the digital economy from a competition perspective and protect consumers. It is difficult to define these new digital enterprises that do not fit snugly into traditional markets. In the European Union, the European Commission described the "structural competition problems" caused by the dynamics of the new markets:

> To give an example, the more people that use a search engine, the better its algorithm gets. The better the algorithm, the better the customer experience and therefore the more people that

use it. And the cycle, in theory, repeats until we have one clear winner in the search engine space . . . Similarly, in the social media space, the more people that use a large social media platform, the more likely you are to join the platform, and not its smaller competitor, thereby entrenching the size differential between platforms (leading to what the European Commission calls *"winner-takes-most' scenarios")*.[127]

These are often referred to as network effects.

A wide range of concerns arises from the power and control of these platforms. The sheer economic strength of a successful platform may enable it to squeeze off smaller competitors, inhibit potential investors from investing in competitors, or simply purchase them. Should a platform like DAC, acting as gatekeeper, be able to charge vendors on the platform a fee and thereby obtain a price advantage by going into competition with them? Or should the gatekeeping platform be able to cull the information it has available about the vendors on the platform and use the information to go downstream into direct competition with the vendor? Should DAC be allowed to go vertical, controlling the entire chain of supplies and workers?

Should a platform be able to keep the data it collects exclusively to itself, thereby securing a competitive advantage, or must it make the data available to competitors? And if it must share, how can it assure privacy to people whose data are now accessed by entities they never contemplated or agreed to?

These and many other issues that policymakers must consider will arise as the paradigm shifts. Some propose to break up the platforms using traditional antitrust approaches. However, many of the traditional definitions do not apply anymore, such as how to define a market and market dominance in such a different, complex ecosystem. Others, as Wheeler et al. explained, "conclude such regulation in the digital era warrants creation of a Digital Platform Agency to establish public interest expectations that promote fair market practices while being agile enough to deal with the rapid pace of digital technology."[128] While the challenges are daunting, some observers are reassured because regulation over dramatic changes in technology has been formulated successfully (from their perspective) in other dimensions of our lives. The Securities and Exchange Commission, for example, protects investors by restricting how and to whom financial information is disclosed. The Food and Drug Administration reviews the manner in which data are collected and the results obtained before approving medications.

Regulators and the regulated will need to work together to develop the standards by which innovations are approved and implemented. For 50 years, government regulators have exerted overweening power over every nut and bolt of the Industrial Age aging care industry. The governmental bureaucracy has been tasked with acting as a traffic cop, standing aside from the actors and controlling decisions and behaviors. The entire industry has had to approach them as supplicants. The regulators have withstood legislative and executive branch efforts to use programs as personal cookie jars while also shielding other governmental branches from the ire of a populace that may want change immediately.

In the new era, regulator and regulated are thrust into a different relationship, not based on uniformity or consistency but on innovation and speed. The regulatory apparatus must move from a focus on processes to a consideration of results. It must establish feedback loops to observe and react immediately to what is learned from the changes that the database tracks. This means moving from bureaucratic, top-down control to responsive relationships in an emergent system. There are models for this. The National Institutes of Health distributes funds to researchers throughout the nation. Their ongoing engagement with the research community and the maintaining of standards during the search for the new approaches to health has led to wonderfully impressive results.

In order to assure that interventions are applied safely and appropriately, regulators will need to monitor new procedures, ensuring that they are not just designed to reduce costs inappropriately or preference certain providers. They will have to determine that procedures are safe, effective, and equitably distributed. The regulatory process itself will have to develop a new culture that responds to data-driven innovation, similar to the Food and Drug Administration and the Centers for Disease Control and Prevention. Data-management agencies such as DAC will evolve into a creative problem-solving arena where innovations can be explored and implemented and will provide exciting venues for the cream of healthcare talent in the United States.

The historic Industrial Age governmental bureaucracies, designed as separate, isolated mini-fiefdoms, will need to be replaced by sophisticated teams of MD/MBAs, MD/PhDs, MD/ITs, and sociologists/MPHs (Masters of Public Health) who work collaboratively with the digital industry to implement innovations.

One of the paramount concerns of the new regulatory structure will be how to share the savings created by less costly aging care between insurers and government funding agencies. With the prospect of enormous savings, it is possible that some states will give multiyear contracts to digital insurer-providers like my DAC, encouraging them to invest in long-term social interventions that will lead to even more efficiencies. Companies will be incentivized to find savings while assuring that government also receives a share of the financial relief. Eventually the industry will mature, and ever more sophisticated algorithms will make equitable sharing relatively uniform in the industry.

Government Regulation of Inside, Outside, and Beside Interventions

The regulation of the Inside interventions described in Chapter 10, such as medications and hip replacements, will remain mostly the business of traditional regulators of healthcare. Those options will continue to fit, albeit with some tensions, within the existing regulatory frameworks. The regulation of Outside interventions, such as fire codes and building standards, were originally designed for nursing homes rather than homecare. They will need to be adapted, balancing safety and independence, as frailty is distributed throughout personal venues in the community.

The most extensive body of new regulations will need to be developed for Beside interventions. Sets of protections will evolve, protecting the relationships among clients and their various providers. Skilled workers will be replaced with less skilled ones, so training requirements will change. Some of what used to be done by physicians will be done by nurse practitioners, as is already happening. Tasks done by nurse practitioners will be handled by nurses, who in turn will give their former responsibilities to aides. Less complex tasks will be delegated to lesser trained people, with professionals retaining only those elements that truly require higher skill. Studies will be conducted to reassure the public that nurse's aides can pass medications with the same efficacy as nurses, and regulations will change accordingly. Not only will it be necessary to protect the clients' safety, but there will also be concerns for workers' protection. As traditional employee roles are blurred by independent contracting, traditional regulations for workers' hours, wages, licensing, and benefits will be recast.

Today, professional practice in the healthcare industry is tightly regulated by laws and licensing agencies. The entire health industry in the United States and all of its segments have been organized around licensing that carefully defines scopes of practice, the boundaries of which are battled over by professional associations and health regulators. These agencies have historically acted as a bulwark against assigning care to less expensive providers. Even if a procedure could be performed safely by lesser trained, less costly professionals, the entrenched regime, eager to retain business, has not permitted the passing down of responsibilities. This system will need to give way. When a change provides a satisfactory service for less cost, the desire to use it is a natural consequence of new technologies interacting with the Law of Interchangeable Interventions.

Eventually, the historic scopes of practice and the related associations of professionals will have to surrender some of their territory. New frameworks to train professionals will replace the old. In some areas, the current specializations of professionals will adapt. In others, an entirely new taxonomy will be overlaid, replacing the old. It will be a challenge to educate people with new skill sets using technical interventions and reeducating them as new interventions appear.

Conclusion

This cannot be a complete compendium of the issues at play, for the aging revolution is occurring on a societal tableau of incredible complexity and scale. As medical interventions fold into social ones it is quite likely that states, with their range of distinct cultures, will assert and control very different approaches to aging.

Given the range of interrelated dynamics at play, the precise form and nature of the aging network and its evolutionary steps are not knowable, but the direction is clear. Incredible advances in infectious medicine in the first half of the 20th century enabled many to survive longer—and obscured from recognition the additional range of societal developments in the second half that also accelerated the longevity revolution. Increasing medicalization of Industrial Age nursing homes and assisted-living residences obscured societal developments that were addressing the range of human dimensions squeezed out of facilities for older adults. The legislative, regulatory and judicial interpretations developed to control the excesses of Gilded Age technologies will evolve again to meet the needs of the Digital Age. Anticipating the coming postindustrial society 50 years ago, sociologist Daniel Bell said, "culture guards the continuity of human experience . . . technology . . . is always disruptive of traditional social forms and creates a crisis for culture."[129] This is the nature of progress. Social developments within underlying society will again enable it to integrate the technological change.

A fundamental hope for the care of older adults is that the accumulation of data and the resulting algorithms are used *for* us. Rather than restricting our freedoms, they may enable us to live with more options and possibilities. The new era of aging will inevitably create legal and ethical challenges, but it must emerge, in some safe format, if we are to absorb the multitudes of older adults who are coming into our midst.

CHAPTER 15

Aging Revealed

The later decades of life often carry with them an accumulation of conditions that destroy the sense of invulnerability prevalent in our younger years. A person's last years may be experienced as ones of quiet desperation and may turn social gatherings into discussions of health complaints, sometimes jokingly referred to as "organ recitals." Niall Williams, in *This Is Happiness*, described his perception of an older man in Ireland prior to such recitals:

> A thing I didn't consider then was that he was over 60 years, getting up, getting down, twisting, bending, flexing, and all in the elasticated parts were matched by aches, clunks and creaks in the skeletal. I pardon my ignorance by the fact that no one spoke of their ailments, there was a now depreciated philosophy of offering it up[130] and half the people of Faha were dead before they thought to complain of pain.[131]

What accounts for this common, earlier custom of silence about the sensations of aging, so perceptively noted by Williams? Perhaps these experiences of older adults were so inextricably tied to later life that there was no understanding of them as mutable, and therefore no purpose in complaining about one's lot in being old? From a long-term historical perspective, the 20th-century unearthing of the causes of the "aches, clunks, and creaks" emancipated us unexpectedly. We suddenly perceived the possibility of being freed of these hindrances. The now familiar "organ recitals" among older people, putting words to discomforts, may actually have been a new possibility for conversation.

Reconsidering Our View of Older Age

Digitization, the vehicle that will accelerate the changes occurring in serving America's aging, has already seeped into many other dimensions of our lives. Those developments are now awakening us to the realization that we are not discussing some theoretical, future reality, but one in which we have already arrived. There will be a tipping point, as aspects of frail aging are identified and detoxified, when people will be able to envision themselves at older chronological age. They will be able to recognize that what have often been viewed as exclusively geriatric health concerns are actually expressions and exacerbations of conditions that have been accumulating throughout their lives. Following the paths of chronic conditions back to their sources leads us earlier and earlier in the life course. "Arteriosclerosis usually starts in the teens and 20s,"[132] for example, and osteoarthritis in the late 40s.[133] Lung function declines,[134] and we begin to lose bone[135] and muscle mass[136] in our 30s. Our sense of balance begins to deteriorate around the age of 25,[137] hearing[138] and sight[139] in our 40s. Recognizing all this helps us realize we are stepping into our futures much sooner than we tend to think. It's a little late to close the barn door in order to avoid all the critters coming into the yard and scratching at the door.

Traditionally, changes in body function have marked the onset of "old age" in people's minds. Now that we are able to identify and explain chronic conditions, to unearth their causes, and to implement new interventions, people are able to live much more comfortably with the changes. Chronic conditions need not thrust people into a new, separate orbit. Or, if people continue to view themselves in an entirely new stage of life, it can now be one that allows them to preserve their individual identities and see their state as one of Benescence.

Made possible by new digital shifts, these new psychological insights about aging will join with a societal transformation, integrating older adults into communities, which will enable them to settle naturally into the rhythm of modern life in the United States. Over steppingstones that may not be visible today, electronic connections will enable us to maintain the social connections that bind us together. The "I am now old" identity has been so powerful that it has too often removed older adults from the wider world.

For some other groups, social developments have already led to integration with society. Their experiences may provide a roadmap as to how rapidly and fundamentally our aging experience will change. I graduated from high school in 1965, a year after the ending of the 18-year birth cohort called the Baby Boomers. Medicare and Medicaid came into law 1 month after my graduation. The Civil Rights Act of 1964 had just passed. Homosexuality was illegal. We were 4 years away from the Stonewall riots. Few physicians or lawyers were female. We were very aware of, and often lived within the boundaries of, our different ethnic enclaves. Religious affiliations tended to organize us into separate groups. Protestants considered Catholics outsiders, although a Catholic president was finally elected in my junior year of high school. Jewish people lived in a parallel, but separate, universe. No person of color had ever been elected to the presidency or vice presidency.

My post–high school years were marked, if not defined, by race, gender, sexual, and religious revolutions. These developments have been variously ascribed to America's ascendant postwar economy, to a reaction to the stultifying 1950s, to the Vietnamese war, to inadequate institutional responses to the Boomer generation's outsized numbers, and to a range of other factors. Whatever the underlying reasons, change came in a fairly consistent pattern. A growing recognition of an inappropriate approach to a given set of people led to defining the group's needs. Protests and demands on behalf of the neglected cohort was followed by pushback against change and, finally, shifts occurred, albeit jaggedly and with residual islands of resistance.

In the space of 15 years, for example, opinion has almost completely reversed about same-sex marriage, from 60% opposed and 31% in favor in 2004 to 61% in favor and 31% opposed as of this writing.[140] How and why did attitudes change so quickly? Charlesworth and Banaji explained that among the other reasons for the rapid changing attitudes is the Widespread Contact Hypothesis:

> [V]ariations in sexual orientations are seen in all parts of society, across rich and poor, males and females, racial and ethnic groups, and all zip codes, states, and countries. Unlike groups defined by race/ethnicity, age, or disability, individuals with different sexual orientations are not as easily segregated. This provides widespread opportunity for positive contact with individuals with different sexual orientations, prompting positive attitude change.[141]

A similar evolution can be seen in attitudes toward women. Although very significant glass ceilings and pay differentials remain, the impact of the women's movement has been profound. Women now make up 36% of doctors in the United States,[142] compared to 5% in 1970.[143] In 2019, women constituted 54.9% of all students in American Bar Association–approved law schools.[144] Only 37.4% of U.S. lawyers are women,[145] but that is an advance over their 4% share in 1970;[146] 59.5% of U.S. college students are female, and in "the next few years, two women will earn a college degree for every man."[147] For the class of 2017–2018, women earned more than half the bachelor's degrees (57.3%), masters degrees (60.1%), and doctoral degrees (53.3%) awarded in the United States.[148] As with the LBGTQ community, women are all around us, sharing all our social and cultural milieux.

Religious identity is also in flux, in large measure because of physical proximity leading to social engagement with others. Research suggests that the rate of interfaith marriage is related to a religious group's size relative to other groups in the same geographic area.[149] How much interaction there is among people of different faiths in large measure determines the acceptance of intermarriage between those people, as represented by its rate of occurrence. For example, as early as 1997, a study found that "the intermarriage rate in dioceses where Catholics were less than 10% of the population was 51%. The intermarriage rate declined steadily until it reached 18% in dioceses where Catholics were a majority of the population."[150] The exponential growth rate of Jewish intermarriage, estimated at 58% among all Jewish people and 71% among non-Orthodox Jewish individuals,[151] has been attributed, among other factors, to "the geographic shift away from areas of high Jewish concentration."[152]

According to analyses reported by the American Enterprise Institute, the primary reason for this changing religious identification and identity is the integration of formerly segregated groups. The author noted,

> Expansions in government service provision and especially increasingly secularized government control of education significantly drive secularization and can account for virtually the entire increase in secularization around the developed world . . . increasingly secularized education serves to directly reduce

religiosity as schools provide a different set of values and life orientations than parents might.[153]

Again, geographic and social engagement with others leads to acceptance, loosening historically locked-in identities.

Ethnic lines are blurring in a manner similar to what has occurred among religious groups in the United States. The Irish, Italian, German, British, Greek, and Slavic ethnic enclaves of the Boomers' early years were blended by postwar suburbanization, among other factors. "By the '90s, only 20% of white Americans had chosen partners from the same ethnic background."[154]

But it is not just geographic proximity that affects the pace of social change. It is also that, under deeper scrutiny, hardline definitions of and boundaries around identity lose significance. Overcoming the historic geographic segregation of race may be less significant than the weakening of the idea of racial identity itself. While the concept of race has always been a social construct without biological meaning,[155] the 2020 U.S. Census reveals that the hard edges of historic separate racial categories it lists do not accurately capture the identities that people hold of themselves.

Historically, the U.S. Census Bureau recognized only one response for race. The 2010 census began to allow people to check more than one box in order "to more accurately capture the profusion of complexity in American demographics."[156] Results in the 2020 census reflected a very fluid color line. There was a doubling of the number of people reporting that they were more than one race.[157] As stated by Richard Alba, "That's not a change in social reality, that's a change in the way social reality is being categorized."[158] David Brooks asserted that "real humans are very quick to adopt multiple and shifting racial identities."[159] Douglas S. Massey, a sociologist at Princeton University, projected that "The whole racial classification system is going to shift in the next few years . . . The off-the-shelf standard American is going to be some kind of blend of Asian, Latino and white."[160]

Facing Our Future Selves

Having grown up experiencing these social movements, Boomers are likely to address the roots of the societal plague of *ageism*, a stereotyped negative attitude toward older adults. Ageism is curious in that, unlike hostility toward people in other groups, it involves turning against one's own future self. It seems almost like an autoimmune disease, where the body's defense mechanisms attack itself. We become alienated against people whom we will eventually come to resemble, despite the fact that the focus of our opprobrium is frail and in need of sympathy and care.

There is research that suggests an explanation for this strange psychological and emotional disconnection with one's own future self. Again, it is influenced by historical institutional segregation, which keeps older adults separate. A person's perceptions about his or her own future self appear to have dramatic impact on the person's willingness to anticipate, plan for, or even to accommodate his or her later years. As articulated by Hal Hershfield, Professor of Marketing, Behavioral Decision Making, and Psychology at UCLA, "when the future self shares similarities with the present self, when it is viewed in vivid and realistic terms, and when it is seen in a positive light, people are more willing to make choices today that benefit them at some point in years to come."[161]

Imagine that a person's life is set on a filmstrip into the future. When the film is stopped at any given point, the future frames or future "selves" lie out ahead. It is hypothesized that we view these future selves much as we do people other than ourselves, or strangers. Again, Hershfield said, "the self is a collection of distinct identities that overlap with one another over time . . . (and) each one of these overlapping selves may share a strong degree of psychological connection with the next one, or they may not."[162] Similar to how we may deal with another person, we deal with our future self. To the degree that those selves are similar to us, attractive or interesting, we may engage, address, accommodate, and share resources with them. Conversely, we may turn our backs, reject, or deny them altogether.

This phenomenon may help to explain the ageism that is rife in the United States. The Industrial Age segregated frailty from the general population in order to bring together resources to address it. In the middle of the epidemiologic Era of Acute and Infectious Disease, the focus was on medical interventions. The historical segregation of frailty in older age from the rest of society distanced them from our younger, less-frail selves and made older people less familiar and less similar to us, particularly because an unfortunate artifact of institutionalized frailty was a concentration of sights and smells that was powerfully off-putting.

We have unintentionally created images of our future selves that are so alien to our current selves that, rather than planning, anticipating and making accommodations for them, we close them out. The images have been so upsetting that we turn away, thinking, "thank goodness that's not me. Let it never be me. And let's not think about this further," setting in motion a cycle of anger, guilt, and shame that can give rise to inhumane behaviors. Those future selves become threats to our present ones. An unfortunate result of segregation of frail older adults is ignorance of the other, leading to dread, denial, fear, and even hatred.

Reintroducing older people more fully into our communities— as will be described in greater detail in the next chapter—so that we see them as multifaceted and interesting human beings, will be an antidote to ageism. As with the LBGTQ, racial, women's, religious, and ethnic groups, this change will not happen until there is more geographic inclusion of frail adults with others in the community. It may in fact happen more quickly than in the previous groups, because for frail people there will be no need to eliminate exclusive academic and social admissions policies, stop the policing of private sexual behavior, force school busing, overcome resistance to subsidized housing in existing neighborhoods, or reverse redlining. As digitized community delivery systems for older adults arrive all around us and replace the aging industrial complex that segregated frail older people, these people will simply remain in place, their younger selves becoming the older members of the neighborhood. After all, they are the indigenous population.

Reduced barriers and burdens will enable them not only to present a much fuller profile to the world, but also to themselves. Limiting, pejorative stereotypes will give way, revealing the expanded achievements and profiles of the group. This can be, for many, the future of older age.

Bernice Neugarten, Professor of Human Development at the University of Chicago, said in 1965 that time itself is socially constructed.

She helped identify "the prescriptive timetables for the ordering of life events."[163] In an article entitled "The Time of our Lives," Kenneth Ferraro explained Neugarten's contribution, writing "people have a sense of the appropriateness of the actions for persons of various ages."[164] That is, we socially construct age. At long last, enabled perhaps by witnessing other social revolutions in their lives, Boomers may become able to loosen and adapt their attitudes toward aging.

Tying previous social expectations to fixed chronological ages is already declining all around us. Eight-hour work weekdays and 40-hour workweeks lose meaning as people work from home. Rather than experiencing decades of employment with one corporation, many people now have multiple careers interspersed with periods of education. The existing time-based framework of work, including full-time and part-time employment and independent contractors, inadequately matches today's realities. Many more people have multiple marriages and multiple families. Fertility and sexual activity have been extended. Overall, peoples' expectations, goals, and activities are decreasingly aligned with chronological age.

The use of generations to measure the passage of time may also fall away under closer scrutiny. As early as 1952, Karl Mannheim questioned the use of equal intervals for defining generations.[165] When he wrote, 30 years was used as a rule of thumb to define a generation. Today, with awareness of the rapid pace of change, some measure generations every 5 years. The worldviews of siblings born even a few years apart may be very different. Clustering people by generation may lose its significance altogether.

This does not mean that chronological age does not exist. Rather, those numbers no longer hold the meaning that they once held, and individuals and communities can impress those years with different meanings. Historic age markers such as 62 and 65 will no longer be the primary indicators of status, rights, and privilege. The extended longevity is way beyond simple youth creep, as expressed by the familiar refrain "70 is the new 60," for that only begins to suggest the changes that are occurring. Stage-of-life theories such as young-old and old-old are also of limited value in describing the fluid dimensions of aging. As chronological rubrics melt away, individuals will be free to recognize and create new attitudes, postures, and roles. Along the way, older adults will recognize the tools available to them and will extend active agency from their earlier years into and throughout their later ones.

Conclusion

The new circumstances will become more widespread as the digital world allows more and more older adults to remain integrated in their communities. Even though tensions will arise because much of the existing aging infrastructure has been based on a relatively static view of chronological age that is no longer matched to the new realities, we will look back and see that much of the way we have looked at aging is simply outdated. Perhaps we will have a fuller sense of the breadth of life throughout all our days. One idea of age has passed, and a new one finds itself revealed among us.

CHAPTER 16

The New Aging

At Home in the Neighborhood

The Law of Interchangeable Interventions has shown us that medical interactions can sometimes be replaced by social ones and that institutionalization often can be replaced by a supported life in the local community. In order for that to occur, individuals and communities will need to develop a new mindset so that they take part directly in how people near them live and age. Local groups must acquire a sense of investment in and influence over the dollars available for aging care. The current system that forces states and communities to go to the federal government to ask for permission for even the tiniest innovation will have to be replaced. The need to localize the responsibility for aging will eventually be recognized, even at the federal level.

Network-Driven Care System

Beyond its impact on healthcare for older adults and traditional institutions, a network-driven care system for aging care employing a lot of helping hands will change the fabric of the communities where that care is delivered. In the last century or so, frail older people have been segregated from community life. If I could look back from the future, perhaps 10 years from now, I would hope to see that we had realized a significant benefit from helping older adults remain in their neighborhoods as they grew older, rather than moving them into unfamiliar settings. As we have seen, it may once have been necessary to segregate an age group from the general population, especially if the separated group was frail, because it was the only way to organize and deliver required care. In the Industrial Age, grouping a cohort together was also the best approach to managing costs. But this exile of older men and women from the neighborhood deprived them of the comfort of familiar surroundings. More than a century ago, social work activist and Nobel Laureate Jane Addams wrote:

> To take away from an old woman whose life has been spent in
> household cares all the foolish little belongings to which her af-
> fections cling and to which her very fingers become accustomed,
> is to take away her last incentive to activity, almost to life itself.[166]

Individual behaviors will need to change, and this will come as a
gradual process as more and more older adults see their contemporaries modeling new behavior. Some such changes have already
happened. In the past century, old age was perceived as a state of
natural decline deserving as gentle a descent as we could provide.
In contrast, today's Baby Boomers—as we have described—are awakening to the possibilities of self-improvement through diet, exercise,
and avoidance of lethal habits like smoking. As they come to realize
these values, the common, unfortunate pattern of hiding one's age-related losses will be eased, if not eliminated. Admitting losses historically has evoked fears of being moved to an institutional setting.
Now, addressing the changes and availing oneself of newly available
interventions in the home will enable people to continue to live on
their own.

Placing a parent in a nursing home, despite his or her resistance,
has heretofore offered families a sense of relief from the financial
burden and direct day-to-day responsibilities of caring for the parent.
That paradigm is also changing as society changes. Nursing homes
and other institutional settings, as they become more medicalized,
will no longer serve as the primary venues for long-term care of frail
older clients. Interventions and eventually government financial support will move to less-expensive options delivered in communities.
And communities themselves will learn to accept solo living as a natural part of the lifespan.

Because the system of segregating older adults still dominates
today's system of care for the frail aging population, it's no wonder
that people often see the prospect of getting old as a terrible time.
Residents in nursing homes exist in a world that exaggerates and
compounds the negative features and losses correlated with older
age, creating a sense that all is slipping away. By contrast, when our
oldest neighbors remain at home in their communities, as I hope
will become the norm, they are more likely to maintain contact with
neighbors of all ages and become a more familiar part of the life cycle.

Life in the community is made even richer by the fact that we don't live in our homes as separate and unconnected islands. We live in neighborhoods. Isolating the oldest generation also denies the rest of us the opportunity to witness how people manage the challenges of aging. As Jane Addams also noted:

> The reminiscences of these old women, their shrewd comments upon life, their sense of having reached a point where they may at last speak freely with nothing to lose because of their frankness, makes them often the most delightful of companions.[167]

Community Living for Older Adults

Community living in older age is not a new system. Older adults were first taken care of in their neighborhoods even before there were poorhouses. In 1915, for example, a group of Jewish women went door to door in their community in Buffalo, NY, to collect money for the care of vulnerable older Jewish adults. They eventually bought a house, hired a housemother, and created what was a sort of orphanage for those of their "landsmen" who had nobody and nothing and were worn out from their labors. Over time, the menfolk of these charitable ladies also became involved. Kosher butchers donated food, Jewish dentists and physicians donated their services, and Jewish businessmen handled the accounts. The ladies, who lived nearby, inspected the home with white gloves, kept up its appearance, and supervised its day-to-day functions. Other religious groups developed similar programs and services for their members all over the country, each taking care of their own. There was minimal government involvement. As the numbers of older adults in the community increased, the residences expanded into larger houses or became infirmaries, but they remained centered in a particular community.

As described in Chapter 6, in 1965 the government began to take over a role in providing assistance to older adults through Medicare and Medicaid. Governmental support reduced the need for funding from the community for many services and, as a consequence, for community leadership. Administrators of institutions became professionals rather than religious or cultural leaders. Priests, rabbis, and social workers were replaced by MBAs. Nursing homes and other congregate settings became highly regulated suppliers of the services for which the government would reimburse them. In response to these new conditions community social networks faded.

It may be that the coming digitized world, with its ability to keep people in their homes, can take us back, in a very modernized way, to the configurations of neighborhoods that we have lost. In the early 1900s we tended to come together to care for our older adults in groups defined by religion, ethnicity, or other common interests. When we federalized aging and healthcare, we removed aging care from the control and involvement of local communities. And now we find ourselves at the threshold of a new age that will have two dominating features: (1) a fast-growing number of people present among us who live longer and carry a burden of chronic conditions for which the Industrial Age health system is rapidly losing effectiveness and (2) the arrival of the Digital Age, providing us with tools to decentralize care for chronic conditions and integrate older adults into community settings. After a long journey through a 20th century dominated by institutions, we are returning to a greatly changed version of where we started.

In order to create such an important new paradigm, multiple adjustments will have to be made. Some of these may come about as our understanding of aging evolves. Many families may worry about the potential isolation of loved ones if they are cared for in their own homes. But, as the number of examples of older adults doing well in their communities increases, it will become clear that this danger is mostly a misperception. In *Going Solo*, sociologist Eric Klinenberg noted that, "during the last half century, our species has embarked on a remarkable social experiment. For the first time in history, great numbers of people . . . have begun settling down as [what he refers to as] singletons."[168] He included a map showing that people living alone constitute 40% of Washington, DC; 45% of Atlanta; 42% of Seattle; and 43% of Minneapolis. He cited "the rising status of women, the communications revolution, mass urbanization, and the longevity revolution" as drivers of this phenomenon.[169]

His findings contradict the common view that living alone somehow is "an unmitigated social problem, a sign of narcissism, fragmentation, and a diminished public life."[170] Not only have those assumptions receded, but new studies also indicate that people living alone may have higher life satisfaction with more personal control, liberation, and self-actualization and that they are more socially engaged.[171] Frail older adults will live in this new society, not the communities of the 1960s and 1970s. Networked communities will rise up to engage frail people in their midst.

When an older adult enters a nursing home, his or her loved ones believe that the person will receive 24-hour care and supervision. In practice, the person remains alone for long periods, often at enormous risk. The physical presence of other people in the building, even though it seems to families to be a benefit in itself, is often unaccompanied by adequate ongoing and thoughtful vigilance or socialization. The resident may be helped very briefly each morning with activities of daily living by nurse's aides who often do not notice even the most obvious changes of status. The staff should observe how the resident is behaving, responding, and eating, and whether he or she is active, dressed, and taking his or her medications, but this level of observation is not always the case. It has taken decades to realize that merely being around others is not an adequate stand-in for careful scrutiny and analysis. We have too often conflated being among others with care.

We recognized the issue of isolation within congregated living decades ago when we redesigned the New Home. In a traditional nursing home, the supervising nurse remains parked at the nursing station and is generally focused on documentation rather than interacting with residents. The nursing station with its camaraderie among the staff tends to attract nurse's aides away from residents' rooms. When not in their rooms, residents often sit clustered together but not interacting, effectively alone in the crowd, in order to increase the efficiency of medication passes, group activities, and meals, all conducted by very narrowly trained staff.

Our New Home, as described previously, eliminated corridors and placed nurse's aides in the middle of clusters of seven or eight rooms. The resident–aide dyad was the critical element of care, but even this innovative improvement depended heavily on minimally trained nurse's aides to notice and report changes. It was a good first try, but it was not enough.

In contrast, the data gathering in an older adult's private home that has been properly outfitted by Digital Aging Care, Inc. (DAC), can provide individually tailored social interactions and communication through social media, personalized screens and devices, and planned visits with meaningful acquaintances and family. DAC can also capture more accurately, more continually, less invasively, and less expensively many indicators of a person's change of status. Robust and ongoing monitoring can result in coordinated and quickly responsive visits from more highly trained and paid caregivers, providing the kind of care that traditional settings promise but often do not deliver. Although the older adult may be living alone, he or she may in fact be less isolated because of a range of social media options and the power of digital monitoring. Responses from caregivers to both physical and emotional needs will be more timely. As families come to see that a parent is not suffering from isolation when he or she is at home, chinks will appear in their belief in the necessity of old congregate settings. When aging is no longer sequestered, a State of Benescence in older age is likely to become a new normal that will give rise to new opportunities to address the final challenge of understanding the behavior of frail older adults in the community.

A person's interest in being with others often evolves with age. The desperate need for intense companionship during adolescence can be very different from the desire for a moment of solitude during the frenetic middle years of work and family life. With older age, social networks often become smaller and more selective. Solitude in older age may offer underrecognized pleasures. The sleep that was so absolute at earlier age may now be caught in snatches. The clear delineations between wakefulness and slumber may fade into shades of consciousness and reflection. Time slows down, uncovering new kinds of awareness. These valuable activities while being alone at older ages were inaccessible and inexplicable in our younger days.

We will learn to identify when and in what circumstances being alone is pleasing, acceptable, unsatisfactory, or harmful to each individual's well-being. We will learn to identify and match resources and interventions appropriately to the ebb and flow of an older adult's experience while living alone. Without forfeiting our concern for the potential emotional, mental, and physical health hazards of being alone, but now also provisioned with the capabilities to support and communicate with a person dwelling alone, we will learn to distinguish the various affective states related to being alone. Societal change (outside) is enabling us to see beyond the old shibboleths of the old maid and the curmudgeon, opening the opportunity to develop nuanced understandings of how being alone works for each individual.

When we have convinced some families, by examples and public information campaigns, that living in the community is a better solution for older adults than institutionalization, and that we have the tools—digital and otherwise—to bring them the care that they need, paradigm shifts to a new, community-based system will begin to occur. But these efforts will not be sufficient and will not bring about change quickly enough in the face of our coming demographic deluge. We must also bring along individual older people and the members of the communities around them. Several developments will come into play. Perhaps the most important will be the activities of organizations like DAC when they arrive to offer new options and incentives to clients. DAC will initiate multiple small-scale initiatives ranging from discounts on healthy food to rewards for compliance with medical treatments in order to determine what will motivate clients to stay healthier and to determine the levers that change behaviors. Such approaches are already employed throughout society, from massive advertising campaigns to strategic posts on social media. DAC will initiate whole batteries of group initiatives that potentially motivate individuals to comply. Their staff will then determine which social interventions change community patterns and mores so that DAC can invest in them on a wider scale.

DAC will be motivated to conduct extensive research by its own financial incentive to replace medical interventions with less expensive social ones. As frail older adults experience the advantages of certain behaviors and treatments, they will gradually awaken to the benefits of specific interventions for themselves and the people with whom they interact. Their families will also see the impact on their loved ones' quality of life.

DAC will also be motivated to encourage adherence to the recommended interventions, an issue that is extremely problematic today. At present, there are minimal systemic approaches to help people continue to comply with the behavioral changes in a prescribed regime of care. Clayton Christensen rated motivation based on the "intensity and immediacy with which clients feel the complications."[172]

An intervention that results in immediate consequences provides ample motivation for adherence. Treatments with deferred consequences are often ignored. As Christianson noted, "there actually are very few business models in healthcare today whose design is . . . to encourage adherence to therapy."[173] He pointed out that there are thousands of billing codes for procedures "but there is not a single billing code for patient adherence or improvement . . ."[174] Personal care physicians in the United States are neither trained nor tasked to support the client as he or she works through the behavioral changes necessary to become more healthy. For example, at a standard annual checkup, even if obesity and its associated problems are notable, the physician may merely suggest weight loss in passing. Yet estimated national medical costs related to obesity range between $147 billion and nearly $210 billion each year.[175] Organizations like DAC will have financial motivation to mine these enormous untapped opportunities by developing systems to help people change their behaviors for their own benefit. They may be able to introduce sweeping changes in the ways that older adults are successfully persuaded to comply with life-saving behaviors.

In addition to persuading individuals to change, it will also be necessary to involve communities in new behaviors toward their older members. An investigation by sociologist Eric Klinenberg provided insight as to the powerful influence of a community's underlying culture. In 1995 there was a severe heat wave in Chicago that resulted in many deaths among older adults. Klinenberg studied two affected communities that had similar demographics for poor individuals[176] yet dramatically different numbers of deaths. In the more successful community there were more well-established social ties. People were engaged with one another. Those types of relationships did not exist in the less-fortunate community, where more people perished.

Klinenberg called the critical factor behind these different outcomes "social infrastructure." He focused on the physical spaces where people linger and gather together, creating a social fabric with mutual support. Similarly, the kind of community that will be most relevant to aging from now on will be the one that is created by people who live within sight and reach of each other. The neighborhood, with the comfort of proximity, is the bedrock on which the future of aging care rests. Fortunately, Americans have a natural inclination to form groups, as noted as early as the 1830s by Alexis de Tocqueville. He found it remarkable how often Americans joined together in various organizations, which he called associations. He said,

> Americans of all ages, all stations of life and all types of disposition constantly form associations . . . Wherever, at the head of some new undertaking, you see the government in France, or a man of rank in England, in the United States you will be sure to find an association.[177]

Such associations often encourage changes in behavior among their members. Perhaps the thinking of René Girard can help to explain how individuals within a community can come to change their behavior, even if it is sometimes very difficult. He suggested that our desires are not actually our original creations, but are borrowed from others. Robert Pogue Harrison described Girard's thinking: "desires are mimetic: I want what others seem to want. Whether I am conscious of it or not (mostly not), I imitate their desires to such a degree that the object itself becomes secondary."[178] Our thinking and behaviors are shaped in unimaginably powerful ways by the contexts in which we find ourselves. Cynthia L. Haven, author of *Evolution of Desire: A Life of René Girard,*[179] summarizing Girard's insights, wrote: "We live derivative lives. We envy and imitate others obsessively, unendingly, often ridiculously."[180] In order to change the behavior of a group, or of an individual within it, the dynamic must change so that new behaviors become desired and expected from one another. As new interventions are proven to be helpful a momentum to change should arise. When the community patterns of smoking, diet, and exercise are changed; when healthy body-image norms are adopted; and when there is common recognition and acceptance of the consistent time and energy necessarily devoted to well-being, those behaviors will be imitated and adapted by older adults.

In their book *Connected*, Nicholas Christakis and James Fowler describe how the "availability of enormous data sets from online sources"[181] has enabled us to create a new science that studies how people and communities within large social networks come to share ideas and behaviors. Mapping relationships between and among people within communities, they discovered that the architecture of peoples' ties to one another are a major factor in the diffusion of innovation. The nature and distance of the relationship determines the strength of the influence. What they call the Three Degrees of Influence Rule demonstrates that influence gradually dissipates when it extends beyond the friend of a friend of a friend.[182] They suggest that the network within the Three Degrees could be manipulated to create cascades of behavioral changes that foster individual and collective health.

So far, however, Americans' natural inclination to reach out to one another and to model behavior for one another has been underdeveloped in relation to frailty because institutions and congregate settings were thought to be the only safe and appropriate venue for care. As frail older adults more often come to reside in the community, more people within their communities will turn to help them, as they help their other neighbors. In the future that I hope for and expect, people will share an unspoken understanding of aging as simply an expected stage of life and will actively engage in enhancing the lives of others in the community. Many communities will join together to reduce expenses, increase accessibility and motivation, reduce anxiety, and find comfort. Of course, not all communities will be supportive. There will be nonfunctional ones, but many communities will engage with one another in refashioned, new ways.

A recognition of a pattern of older adults finding one another geographically and acting together was first captured in the 1980s by the urban planner Michael Hunt, who called such developments Naturally Occurring Retirement Centers, or NORCs. The phenomenon has been defined geographically as either building based (vertical), neighborhood based (horizontal), or rural. There have been any number of federal and state programs to support NORCs, generally with funding for social services that has so far been inadequate to meet the needs of frail older people. Now, with the coordination of interventions possible with digitization, NORCs can become core associations for aging care in the United States.

Another example of a community development is provided by the concept of cohousing that was developed in Denmark in the 1960s and introduced to the United States by architects Kathryn McCamant and Charles Durrett.[183] Cohousing is an arrangement where people build private homes clustered around shared spaces. They are designed for neighbors to benefit from cost savings, shared amenities and services, and a sense of community where people have expectations of one another. Previously, senior cohousing groups might have become overwhelmed by care needs as the group ages in place. A group like DAC, however, can take over what might have been overwhelming unrealistic expectations and duties among friends, allowing a neighbor to continue in a more reasonable supplementary role and maintaining the social engagement of the group. With DAC's orchestration of frailty care, the potential for cohousing among social cohorts would be greatly strengthened.

The sharing economy can also be seen as a new type of community association made possible by digitization that can become useful for older adults. For example, Airbnb works because it developed a system that enables clients to trust strangers sufficiently to rent a place they own. Similarly, crowdsourcing can be used to draw in people to care for older neighbors because they can obtain payment for providing services ranging from companionship to meals to simply serving as a contact called by DAC to check in when there are indicators of change.

This kind of network already exists, but its enormous potential for caring for older people has been barely tapped. Nextdoor, founded in 2008, has enabled individuals to connect with others living nearby, to talk about what's going on in their neighborhood, and to help one another. It has helped coordinate information and activity in hundreds of thousands of neighborhoods. In 2021, Nextdoor went public through a merger with a special purpose acquisition company (SPAC) in a deal worth $4.3 billion,[184] enabling it to be flexible in its program development. These types of organizations could provide venues that could be charged with determining personal needs and appropriate interventions.

Communities will still look for leadership to help in caring for older adults in their midst, but their leaders will no longer be oriented to supporting only institutional models. The 80 million Millennials, born from 1980 to 2000, are the generation that will be taking up the care of much of the country's currently aging population, and they are the ideal group for the new digital paradigm. David Burstein described the Millennials as practical idealists. Many are resourceful, civic-minded, and optimistic about their own economic futures.[185] Burstein writes, "The Millennial mindset is particularly appropriate and sustainable when it comes to addressing these kinds of intricate, generation-long challenges."[186] They will come to the fore with their own orientation towards re-creating aging for their grandparents and will be open to the way DAC does business. They will also understand that it may take a lifetime to effect change. They don't depend on government to take the lead, and they will start with small local efforts to unleash new interdependent forms of community.

Anthropologist Margaret Mead put this development in a larger societal context. In 1970, she predicted the shifting directions from which generational power would flow. She explained that in transitional models, the cultural transmission is from older to younger members of society. It is past-oriented. As the model breaks down, as it did with the youth culture of the 1960s and 1970s, for example, there is a short-lived, transitional period during which cultural transition is shared. It becomes present-oriented. Finally, Mead predicted the cultural transition power would emanate from the child and be future-oriented. This later development has arrived, as she predicted, driven by the digital revolution.[187] This will be the Boomer generation's healthcare experience: from big institutions, hospitals, and nursing homes, to a proliferation of residential and early community alternatives, to networks, the latter driven by their children.

As communities move toward integrating older adults' interests into mainstream community life, their civic organizations will evolve. Leadership will come to understand the threat of chronic conditions and the advantages of digital programs and begin to facilitate community support networks. Lay community leaders will recognize that they can no longer address their population's challenges through old institutional approaches that require more and more funds just to stay in existence. They will no longer try to reshape traditional agencies but will start fresh. Rather than building facilities to cocoon older adults, they will work to engage them with systems and programs that support and enhance health and well-being.

Although this book traces a linear developmental path, it is unlikely that our system of caring for those in their later years will develop in this precise order or with these particular results. There are simply too many moving parts and too many different participants to predict an exact course.

Each community's pace of adopting new ways to address the dislocation of its older members will be determined by its inventory of assets, the order of changes, and—most critically—the vision of its leadership. The sequence of innovations that are adopted or that arrive suddenly because of technological, social, or regulatory shifts will affect the ability of communities to adapt efficiently and productively. Community leaders may engage with or turn their backs on images of new delivery systems of frailty interventions. Some leaders will persist in plowing money into keeping the old institutional structures in place. When the value of those assets dissipates, their community will become hamstrung, unable to address adequately the health challenges facing their frail older citizens.

The distinctions between local and national efforts will be blurred. The aggregating power of digital technology will enable us to collect massive amounts of data to design and operate a universe of digital interventions. Just as this information flows from the individual to the center for processing and management, so too it flows from the center back to each individual on his or her block. DAC will know where its subscribers live and what resources are available to each one. We will be able to age locally while enjoying the supports of a national-scale care system for older adults. The small neighborhood block and the whole nation can occupy the same space in an entirely new way. The person whose physical world is bounded by what he or she can see from the front window also lives in the boundless world of digital connections. A universe of interventions is concentrated on one very old individual who happily remains in the setting he or she likes best. Now, instead of disappearing into a facility, this person, even when very frail, will stay on the block longer, perhaps even for the rest of his or her life. More older neighbors will be in sight or in reach, where younger people can visit and learn from them. The oldest members of the micro-community will be able to see themselves as part of a world full of variety and stimulation.

We will age in our neighborhoods because it will become the best choice, affirming that every age has a place in our daily lives. All the changes that are coming, from the end of the industrial model of aging care, to the rise of digital solutions in aging care, to the re-integration of older adults into neighborhood life, will create new opportunities.

This may be an antidote to the present concern about the malaise of community. Robert Putnam, in *Bowling Alone*,[188] described in exacting detail the loss of community relationships and institutions. In *The Vanishing Neighbor*,[189] Marc J. Dunkelman explained how local community relationships, which he calls "the middle ring" of our acquaintances, have shrunk. Neither author offered a way out or a way back to strong, vibrant community. Perhaps the underlying foundation for community was economic all along. Locals bought and sold from one another. Stores, restaurants, schools, services, farm produce, and healthcare were all local. National and international supply chains and networks disrupted that. And perhaps frail aging is the vehicle that returns us to economic interdependence and to relationships with one another. The nature and scale of frailty in communities may force us to engage with one another. We are about to re-create community from the ground up. While the chip will provide information and fantastic technological supports, it will be the human element that will enable the community to sustain frail older adults in its midst and make older age a time of life that is important for all ages to know. If Alexis de Tocqueville were to arrive back in the United States in 2030, he would say that he is not surprised; the Township Society that he described in 1831 is alive and well. It is our opportunity to make it so.

Why, if it is possible to improve the global health of older adults, haven't we already done so? Is this vision a vain hope? I contend that it is not impossible, but that we have not already created a new world for our older population because before now we did not understand aging. We didn't understand aging because it was too new. The evolution of aging itself and our understanding of aging in the past century has brought us to a position from which we now realize that aging is not a disease and that the conditions and diseases that are common in older age are as manageable as at any other stage of life. They are not inherent in aging itself, and there is no reason that an older adult cannot maintain a better State of Benescence than we have known.

It is urgent that we compress the time it will take a new understanding of health in older age to sink in and produce meaningful action. Fifty long years passed between the determination that cigarette smoking causes lung cancer and the last days of the smoking culture. Our aging population deserves a faster result. Fortunately, several factors have converged that can make a revolution in late-life health behavior more possible than it has been before now:

1. The new understanding that older age is a time when good health is as normal as at any other age, not a stage of inevitable decrepitude;

2. The knowledge that at any age, including older age, one derives health-promoting benefits from exercise, good diet, socialization, good sleep habits, and the avoidance of unhealthy behaviors like smoking and excessive drinking;

3. The fact that many more older adults see each other out in the world today and can see what good health at advanced ages looks like; and

4. The growing appreciation that older age is not a disaster with conditions that are beyond one's control, but a time of life to be navigated and managed like any other age.

Aging is much more flexible, much more open to possibility, much more fluid than we realize. Our current picture of aging is a concept, not an immutable fact. It is influenced both by the environment and the imprint of our own experiences. It is time that we open aging to its full potential.

I have seen such transformations in the past. The first time was when we packed everyone from the old downtown nursing home in Buffalo onto buses and ambulances and moved them to the New Home. They went from a crowded, batch-processed, airless existence, to roomy, quiet, private, individualized living. By dinner on the very first day our poor, tattered residents were already transformed into gentle people quietly chatting and dining, appearing not much different from the clientele in the restaurant down the way. Underneath were the same needs for support in eating, toileting, dressing, and orientation, but their presentation to the world had changed profoundly. The shock of that transformation was an experience that I would see repeatedly throughout 30 more years in the aging field.

Over and over, through all the various settings and programs we designed, we continually uncovered previously hidden competencies. But we never got to the bottom of the pile of coverings. We always felt that there was more we could do to change the lives of older adults.

Beyond its impact on healthcare for older adults and traditional institutions, a network-driven care system employing a lot of helping hands will change the fabric of the communities where that care is delivered. As we have seen, frail older adults have been segregated from community life in the last century or so. When many more of them are living comfortably in their homes, as they prefer, and new interventions are keeping them safe and in a State of Benescence, a DAC workforce will come and go every day almost like the members of a large family. The aides will be a familiar sight, and they will know to open the windows and raise the blinds to reduce the separation of the person from his or her street.

Conclusion

We now have the capability to effect transformative change in the lifespan. Dramatically increased longevity offers many more decades of life. The map of those years has been uncharted because so few have traversed it before. It is time to begin to upgrade the pathway. The power of the Law of Interchangeable Interventions can have a much broader impact on frail older adults in the community than the New Home did on nursing care. As they age, Boomers will awaken to a different era, ready for them to explore. Millions will experience a natural and fulfilling extension of their lives.

References

1. Omran, A.R. Shifts in mortality and disease patterns. The epidemiologic transition: A theory of the epidemiology of population change. *The Milbank Memorial Fund Quarterly.* 1971;49(4, pt. 1, October). https://doi:10.1111/j.1468-0009.2005.00398.x.

2. Rogers, L.T. America's age profile told through population pyramids. United States Census Bureau. June 23, 2016. https://www.census.gov/newsroom/blogs/random-samplings/2016/06/americas-age-profile-told-through-population-pyramids.html.

3. Roberts, A., Ogunwole, S., Blakeslee, L., & Rabe, M. A snapshot of the fastest growing older population. United States Census Bureau. October 30, 2018. https://www.census.gov/library/stories/2018/10/snapshot-fast-growing-us-older-population.html.

4. Omran.

5. Olshansky, S.J., & Ault, A.B. The fourth stage of the epidemiologic transition: The age of delayed degenerative diseases. *The Milbank Memorial Fund Quarterly.* 1986;64(3), 355–391.

6. Solomon, L.D. *The quest for human longevity: Science, business, and public policy.* New York: Routledge; 2006, 2.

7. Roizen, M. *RealAge: Are you as young as you can be?* New York, HarperCollins; 1999.

8. Fogel, R.W. "Economic growth, population theory, and physiology: The bearing of long-term processes on the making of economic policy." Nobel Lecture (December 9, 1993). University of Chicago, Center for Population Economics. https://www.nobelprize.org/uploads/2018/06/fogel-lecture.pdf.

9. Fries, J.F. Aging, natural death, and the compression of morbidity. *New England Journal of Medicine.* 1980;303(3; August), 130.

10. Omran.

11. Naisbitt, J. *Megatrends: Ten new directions transforming our lives.* New York: Warner; 1982.

12. Fogel, R. Robert Fogel quotes. BrainyQuote.com, https://www.brainyquote.com/quotes/robert_fogel_566619.

13. Hershfield, H.E. Future self-continuity: How conceptions of the future self-transform intertemporal choice. *Annals of the New York Academy of Science.* October 24, 2011. https://doi: 1111/j.1749-6632.2011.06201.x.

14. National Institute on Aging, National Institutes of Health. Why population aging matters: A global perspective. 2017; publication no. 07-6134. https://www.nia.nih.gov/sites/default/files/2017-06/WPAM.pdf

15. Vollset, S.E., Goren, E., Yuan, C.-w., Cao, J., Smith, A.E., Hsiao, T., et al. Fertility, mortality, migration, population scenarios for 195 countries and territories from 2017 to 2100: A forecasting analysis for the Global Burden of Disease study. *The Lancet.* 2020 [396(10258)]. https://doi.org/10.1016/S0140-6736(20)30677-2.

16. Chandran, N. Foreigners could ease Japan's labor shortage, but Tokyo prefers robots. *CNBC.* March 15, 2018. https://www.cnbc.com/2018/03/09/foreigners-could-ease-japans-labor-shortage-but-tokyo-prefers-robots.html.

17. Cave, D., Bubola, E., & Sang-Hun, C. Long slide looms for world population, with sweeping ramifications. *The New York Times.* May 23, 2021.

18. Lufkin, B. What the world can learn from Japan's robots. *BBC.* February 6, 2020. https://www.bbc.com/worklife/article/20200205-what-the-world-can-learn-from-japans-robots.

19. Hahn, A., & Tarver, J. 2022 student loan debt statistics: Average loan debt. *Forbes Advisor.* June 9, 2022. https://www.forbes.com/advisor/student-loans/average-student-loan-statistics/.

20. Zimmerman, J. What is college worth? *The New York Review of Books.* 2020;68(11; July 2). https://www.nybooks.com/articles/2020/07/02/what-is-college-worth/.

21. Student Loan Hero. A look at the shocking student loan debt statistics for 2022. *Student Loan Hero.* July 29, 2022. https://studentloanhero.com/student-loan-debt-statistics/

22. Zimmerman, 37.

23. Orszag, P.R., & Kane, T.J. Higher education spending: The role of Medicaid and the business cycle. Brookings Institution. September 19, 2003. https://www.brookings.edu/research/higher-education-spending-the-role-of-medicaid-and-the-business-cycle/.

24. Orszag & Kane.

25. Levy, G. Increases in Medicaid spending come at the expense of higher education: Study. *U.S. News & World Report.* May 1, 2018. https://www.usnews.com/news/national-news/articles/2018-05-01/increases-in-medicaid-spending-come-at-the-expense-of-higher-education-study.

26. Gleckman, H. The federal government will spend half its budget on older adults in ten years. *Forbes.* February 1, 2019. https://www.forbes.com/sites/howardgleckman/2019/02/01/the-federal-government-will-spend-half-its-budget-on-older-adults-in-ten-years/?sh=3fbd4dbc56b6.

27. Roos, D., Jones, D.T., & Womack, J.P. *The machine that changed the world: The story of lean production.* Berkeley, CA, Free Press; 2007.

28. Ogle, R. *Smart world: Breakthrough creativity and the new science of ideas.* Boston, Harvard Business School Press; 2007.

29. Ogle, p. 2.

30. Firozi, P. The Health 202: States scramble to head off future Medicaid shortfalls. *The Washington Post.* February 21, 2019.

31. Housing for the Elderly (Section 202). 2020 Summary Statement and Initiatives, 28-FY16CJ. https://www.hud.gov/sites/documents/28-fy16cj-housing elderly.pdf.

32. Ahmad, F.B., Cisewski, J.A., Anderson, R.N. Provisional mortality data—United States, 2021. National Library of Medicine, *Morbidity and Mortality Weekly Report.* 2022;71(17, April 29), 597–600. http://dx.doi.org/10.15585/mmwr.mm7117e1.

33. World Health Organization. Measuring health and disability, June 16, 2012. https://www.who.int/standards/classifications/international-classification-of-functioning-disability-and-health/who-disability-assessment-schedule.

34. World Health Organization. International classification of functioning, disability and health, 2001. https://www.who.int/standards/classifications/international-classification-of-functioning-disability-and-health.

35. Nader, R. *Unsafe at any speed*. New York, Grossman; 1965.

36. Aronson, L. U.S. hospitals ignore improving elder care. That's a mistake. *STAT News*. November 16, 2018. https://www.statnews.com/2018/11/16/hospitals-downplay-elder-care/.

37. Genworth. Costs of care: Trends and insights; 2022. https://www.genworth.com/aging-and-you/finances/cost-of-care/cost-of-care-trends-and-insights.html.

38. State of the Union: Budget. USAFacts. https://usafacts.org/state-of-the-union-2021/budget/

39. Ortman, J.M., Velkoff, V.A., Hogan, H. An aging nation: The older population in the United States. United States Census Bureau. May 2014, report P25-1140. https://www.census.gov/library/publications/2014/demo/p25-1140.html.

40. Brandon, E. How much will you get from Social Security? *U.S. News and World Report*. January 21, 2020.

41. Nova, A. Baby Boomers face more risk to their retirement than previous generations. *CNBC*. November 7, 2018. https://www.cnbc.com/2018/11/07/one-third-of-baby-boomers-had-nothing-saved-for-retirement-at-age-58-.html.

42. Stanford Center on Longevity. Seeing our way to financial security in the age of increased longevity. Stanford Center on Longevity. October 2018. https://longevity.stanford.edu/seeing-our-way-to-financial-security-in-the-age-of-increased-longevity-2/.

43. Levey, N.N. 100 million people in America are saddled with health care debt. *Kaiser Health News*. June 16, 2022.

44. Carroll, A.E. Out-of-pocket costs put Americans into medical debt. *New York Times*. July 8, 2022, p. A21.

45. Levey.

46. Lindquist, L.A., Ramirez-Zohfeld, V., Forcucci, C., Sunkara, P., & Cameron, K.A. Overcoming reluctance to accept home-based support from an older adult perspective. *Journal of the American Geriatric Society*. 66 (9; August 29, 2018). https://doi:10.1111/jgs.15526.

47. Medina, L., Sabo, S., & Vespa, J. Living longer: Historical and projected life expectancy in the United States, 1960 to 2060. Population estimates and projections. P25-1145, issued February 2020. https://www.census.gov/content/dam/Census/library/publications/2020/demo/p25-1145.pdf.

48. Mishra, S. Does modern medicine increase life expectancy: Quest for the Moon Rabbit? *Indian Heart Journal*. 2016;68(January–February), 19–27.

49. Sloan, M., Premkumar, A., & Sheth, N. Projected volume of primary total joint arthroplasty in the U.S., 2014 to 2030. *Journal of Bone and Joint Surgery*. 2018;100(17; September 5), 1455–1460.

50. Colonius, E., & Kover, A. Techno sapiens: The convergence of human and technology. *Fortune*. July 8,1996. https://money.cnn.com/magazines/fortune/fortune_archive/1996/07/08/214357/index.htm.

51. Cole, D. Repairing and replacing body parts: What's next. *National Geographic*. April 18, 2013. https://www.nationalgeographic.com/science/article/130415-replacement-body-parts-longevity-medicine-health-science.

52. Wilson, E.O. *The meaning of human existence*. New York, Liveright; 2014, 14.

53. OXO (kitchen utensils brand), Wikipedia, https://en.wikipedia.org/wiki/OXO_(kitchen_utensils_brand).

54. Chari, A.V., Engberg, J., Ray, K.N., & Mehrotra, A. The opportunity costs of the informal elder-care in the United States: New estimates from the American time use survey. *Health Services Research*. 2015;50(3; June 2015). https://doi:10.1111/1475-6773.12238.

55. Waddill, K. Top chronic diseases behind payer spending and how to prevent them. *Healthpayer Intelligence*. June 26, 2020. https://healthpayerintelligence.com/news/top-chronic-diseases-behind-payer-spending-and-how-to-prevent-them.

56. Span, P. In the nursing home, empty beds and quiet halls. *New York Times*. September 28, 2018. https://www.nytimes.com/2018/09/28/health/nursing-homes-occupancy.html.

57. Walsh, J.D. The coming disruption. *New York Magazine*. May 11, 2020. https://nymag.com/intelligencer/2020/05/scott-galloway-future-of-college.html?regwall-newsletter-signup=true.

58. Walgreens Newsroom. 2019. Walgreens Boots Alliance and Microsoft establish strategic partnership to transform healthcare delivery. https://news.microsoft.com/2019/01/15/walgreens-boots-alliance-and-microsoft-establish-strategic-partnership-to-transform-health-care-delivery/; also, walgreensbootsalliance.com.

59. McLymore, A. Walmart, UnitedHealth to offer preventive healthcare program for seniors, Reuters. September 7, 2022. https://www.reuters.com/business/health care-pharmaceuticals/walmart-unitedhealth-offer-joint-program-preventive-healthcare-seniors-2022-09-07/.

60. Hirsch, L. CVS makes $8 billion bet on the return of the house call. *The New York Times*. September 5, 2022. https://www.nytimes.com/2022/09/05/business/cvs-signify-health.html.

61. Terlep, S. CVS agrees to buy home-healthcare company signify for $8 billion. *Wall Street Journal*. September 5, 2022. https://www.wsj.com/articles/cvs-announces-deal-to-acquire-home-healthcare-company-signify-11662411855.

62. Peterson, H. Amazon's delivery business reveals staggering growth as it's on track to deliver 3.5 billion packages globally this year. *Business Insider*. December 19, 2019. https://www.businessinsider.in/business/news/amazons-delivery-business-reveals-staggering-growth-as-its-on-track-to-deliver-3-5-billion-packages-globally-this-year/articleshow/72890618.cms?fromNewsdog=1&utm_source=NewsDog&utm_medium=referral.

63. Walmart. Walmart releases 2017 annual report, proxy statement, global responsibility report and global ethics and compliance program update. April 20, 2007. https://corporate.walmart.com/newsroom/2017/04/20/walmart-releases-2017-annual-report-proxy-statement-global-responsibility-report-and-global-ethics-and-compliance-program-update.

64. Covington, C. Breaking down the silos of mental and physical healthcare. ALM Benefits Pro. 2018. https://www.benefitspro.com/2018/07/06/breaking-down-the-silos-of-mental-and-physical-hea/?slreturn=2022110614023.

65. Horvitz-Lennon, M., Kilbourne, A.M., & Pincus, H.A. From silos to bridges: Meeting the general healthcare needs of adults with severe mental illnesses. *Health Affairs*. 2006;25(3), 659-669. https://doi:10.1377/hlthaff.25.3.659.

66. Interlandi, J. Experts say we have the tools to fight addiction. So why are more Americans overdosing than ever? *New York Times*. June 24, 2022, 5.

67. Interlandi.

68. Interlandi.

69. McChrystal, S. *Team of teams: New rules of engagement for a complex world*. New York: Penguin; 2015.

70. McChrystal, p. 194.

71. McChrystal, p. 145.

72. McChrystal, p. 243.

73. Centers for Disease Control and Prevention. U.S. burden of Alzheimer's disease, related dementias to double by 2060 (September 20, 2018). https://www.cdc.gov/media/releases/2018/p0920-alzheimers-burden-double-2060.html.

74. Agespace; 2022. Dementia life expectancy: Progression and stages after diagnosis. https://www.agespace.org/dementia/life-expectancy.

75. Span, P. To prevent dementia, go for an eye exam. *The New York Times*. July 5, 2022, D3.

76. Weaver, D. Alzheimer's might not actually be a brain disease, expert says. *Science Alert*. 2022 (September 20). https://www.sciencealert.com/alzheimers-might-not-actually-be-a-brain-disease-expert-says.

77. Dooley, B., & Ueno, H. Japan looks to surveillance to keep an eye on its elderly. *The New York Times*. February 8, 2022.

78. Bryson, B. *One summer: America 1927*. New York, Doubleday; 2013. 379–380.

79. Chapin, C.F. How did healthcare get to be such a mess? *The New York Times*. June 19, 2017.

80. Chapin, C.F. (2015). *Ensuring America's health*. New York, Cambridge University Press; 2015.

81. Chapin, p. 4.

82. Chapin, p. 5.

83. Chapin.

84. Christensen, C.M., Grossman, J.H., & Hwang, J. *The innovators prescription: A disruptive solution for healthcare*. New York, McGraw-Hill; 2009, 167.

85. Chapin, p. 7.

86. McGuire, T.G., Newhouse, J.P., & Sinaiko, A.D. An economic history of Medicare Part C. *The Milbank Quarterly*. 2011;89(2; June), 289–332.

87. Kent, J. UnitedHealthcare invests over $400M in social determinants of health. *Healthpayer Intelligence*. April 2, 2019. https://healthpayerintelligence.com/news/unitedhealthcare-invests-over-400m-in-social-determinants-of-health.

88. Michas, F. Number of all hospital beds in the U.S. 1975 to 2019. *Statista*. February 9, 2021. https://www.statista.com/statistics/185860/number-of-all-hospital-beds-in-the-us-since-2001/.

89. United States Hospital Beds. *Trading Economics*, 2022. United States Hospital Beds - 2022 Data - 2023 Forecast - 1960-2021 Historical - Chart (tradingeconomics.com)

90. Roberts, N.F. The history of hospice: A different kind of health "care." *Forbes*. June 22, 2018, https://www.forbes.com/sites/nicolefisher/2018/06/22/the-history-of-hospice-a-different-kind-of-health-care/?sh=3ad46e15660c.

91. Newman, L. Elisabeth Kübler-Ross. *British Medical Journal*. 329 [7466 (2004)], 627. https://www.ncbi.nlm.nih.gov/pmc/articles/PMC516672/.

92. Centers for Medicare and Medicaid Benefits. *Medicare hospice benefits*. https://www.medicare.gov/Pubs/pdf/02154-medicare-hospice-benefits.pdf.

93. Chidambara, P. Over 200,000 residents and staff in long-term care facilities have died from COVID-19. Kaiser Family Foundation, February 3, 2022. https://www.kff.org/policy-watch/over-200000-residents-and-staff-in-long-term-care-facilities-have-died-from-covid-19/.

94. Spanko, A. CMS to adjust PDPM "as quickly as possible" amid evidence of $1.7B nursing home payment increase. *Skilled Nursing News*. April 9, 2021. https://skillednursingnews.com/2021/04/cms-to-adjust-pdpm-as-quickly-as-possible-amid-evidence-of-1-7b-nursing-home-payment-increase/.

95. Stockman, F., Richtel, M., Ivory, D., & Smith, M. "They're death pits": Virus claims at least 7,000 lives in U.S. nursing homes. *The New York Times*. April 17, 2020.

96. Gleckman, H. The grim post-COVID-19 future for nursing homes. *Forbes*. May 4, 2020. https://www.forbes.com/sites/howardgleckman/2020/05/04/the-grim-post-covid-19-future-for-nursing-homes/?sh=232e3dd82448.

97. New York City Comptroller. Report of the New York City comptroller on the sale of two deed restrictions governing property located at 45 Rivington Street. https://comptroller.nyc.gov/reports/report-of-the-new-york-city-comptroller-on-the-sale-of-two-deed-restrictions-governing-property-located-at-45-rivington-street/.

98. Hobbs, A. Mayor's revisions to deed restriction process "not enough," community says. *dna info*. July 13, 2016. https://www.dnainfo.com/new-york/2016 0713/lower-east-side/mayors-revisions-deed-restriction-process-not-enough-community-says/.

99. Mount Sinai plans to open behavioral health center in Rivington House Building. *The Lo-Down*. December 18, 2018. https://www.thelodownny.com/leslog/2018/12/mount-sinai-plans-to-open-behavioral-health-center-in-rivington-house-building.html.

100. Baxter, A. Where the home health aide shortage will hit hardest by 2025. *Home Health Care News*. May 5, 2018. https://homehealthcarenews.com/2018/05/where-the-home-health-aide-shortage-will-hit-hardest-by-2025/.

101. Franck, T. Social Security trust funds now projected to run out of money sooner than expected due to Covid, Treasury says, *CNBC*. August 31, 2021. https://www.cnbc.com/2021/08/31/social-security-trust-funds-set-to-be-depleted-sooner-than-expected.html.

102. Waggoner, J. 9 ways to strengthen Social Security: The truth about its current status and options for boosting its future stability. AARP, March 1, 2022. https://www.aarp.org/retirement/social-security/info-2022/benefits-current-status-future-stability.html.

103. Hamel, L., Lopes, L. Kirzinger, A., Sparks, G., Kearney, A., Stockes, M., & Brodie, M. Public opinion on prescription drugs and their prices. KFF Health

Tracking Poll September 23–October 4, 2021. Kaiser Family Foundation. October 18, 2021. https://www.kff.org/health-costs/poll-finding/public-opinion-on-prescription-drugs-and-their-prices/.

104. Hammond, J., & Gray, G. The future of America's entitlements: What you need to know about the Medicare and Social Security Trustees reports. *American Action Forum*. September 1, 2021. https://www.americanactionforum.org/research/the-future-of-americas-entitlements-what-you-need-to-know-about-the-medicare-and-social-security-trustees-reports-4/#ixzz7POdntyue.

105. Spanko, A. Medicaid's share of nursing home revenue, resident days hits record high as Medicare drops to historic low. *Skilled Nursing News*. December 11, 2019. https://skillednursingnews.com/2019/12/medicaids-share-of-nursing-home-revenue-resident-days-hits-record-high-as-medicare-drops-to-historic-low/.

106. Osterland, A. Aging Baby Boomers raise the risk of a long-term care crisis in the U.S. *CNBC*. November 8, 2021. https://www.cnbc.com/2021/11/08/aging-baby-boomers-raise-the-risk-of-a-long-term-care-crisis-in-the-us.html.

107. Genworth; 2022. Median cost of nursing home, assisted living and home care. https://www.genworth.com.

108. AARP. Nearly half of Americans 55+ have no retirement savings. AARP. March 28, 2019. https://www.aarp.org/retirement/retirement-savings/info-2019/no-retirement-money-saved.html.

109. BarnesWendling CPAs, Inc. Retirement planning for Baby Boomers: It's not too late to save. BarnesWendling. December 5, 2021. https://www.barneswendling.com/retirement-planning-for-baby-boomers-its-not-too-late/.

110. Genworth; 2022. Cost of care survey. https://www.genworth.com/aging-and-you/finances/cost-of-care.html.

111. Rowe, J.W. The U.S. eldercare workforce is falling further behind. *National Aging*. 2021;1(April 12), 327–329. https://doi.org/10.1038/s43587-021-00057-z.

112. Berklan, J.M. Nursing home occupancy woes worse than popularly reported, industry expert says," *McKnight's Long-term Care News*. December 15, 2021. https://www.mcknights.com/news/nursing-home-occupancy-woes-worse-than-popularly-reported-industry-expert-says/.

113. Berklan.

114. AHCA/NCAL. Financial challenges continue to affect nursing homes, emphasizing need for higher Medicaid reimbursement rates. American Health Care Association and the National Center for Assisted Living. October 14, 2020. https://www.ahcancal.org/News-and-Communications/Press-Releases/Pages/Financial-Challenges-Continue-To-Affect-Nursing-Homes,-Emphasizing-Need-For-Higher-Medicaid-Reimbursement-Rates.aspx#.

115. Gleckman, H. The grim post-COVID-19 future for nursing homes. *Forbes*. May 4, 2020. https://www.forbes.com/sites/howardgleckman/2020/05/04/the-grim-post-covid-19-future-for-nursing-homes/?sh=232e3dd82448116.

116. Osterland, A. Aging Baby Boomers raise the risk of a long-term care crisis in the U.S. *CNBC*. November 8, 2021. https://www.cnbc.com/2021/11/08/aging-baby-boomers-raise-the-risk-of-a-long-term-care-crisis-in-the-us.html.

117. Manjoo, F. (2022). The rise of big tech may just be starting. *The New York Times*. February 17, 2022.

118. Manjoo.

119. Manjoo, F. (2022). It's scary how dominant Apple has become. But how scary? *The New York Times*. March 31, 2022.

120. Phillips Sawyer, L. U.S. antitrust law and policy in historical perspective. Working Paper 19-110. http://www.hbs.edu/ris/Publication%20Files/19-110_e21447 ad-d98a-451f-8ef0-ba42209018e6.pdf.

121. Wheeler, T., Verveer, P., & Kimmelman, G. The need for regulation of big tech beyond antitrust. Techtank, Brookings Institution. September 23, 2020. https://www.brookings.edu/blog/techtank/2020/09/23/the-need-for-regulation-of-big-tech-beyond-antitrust/.

122. Zuboff, S. *The age of surveillance capitalism: The fight for a human future at the new frontier of power.* New York: Public Affairs; 2019.

123. Zuboff, p. 8.

124. Zuboff, p. 11.

125. Zuboff, p. 11

126. Zuboff, p. 21.

127. McCannFitzgerald. What the tech is going on with digital markets and antitrust/competition law? *McCannFitzgerald Knowledge*. November 27, 2020. https://www.mccannfitzgerald.com/knowledge/antitrust-competition/what-is-going-on-with-digital-markets-and-antitrust-competition-law.

128. Wheeler, T., Verveer, P., & Kimmelman, G. The need for regulation of big tech beyond antitrust. Techtank, Brookings Institution. September 23, 2020. https://www.brookings.edu/blog/techtank/2020/09/23/the-need-for-regulation-of-big-tech-beyond-antitrust/.

129. Bell, D. *The Winding Passage: Essays and Sociological Journeys 1960–1980.* New York: Basic Books; 1970, 7.

130. Berg, T.V. What does it really mean to "offer it up"? *Catholic Digest*. December 5, 2017. https://www.catholicdigest.com/from-the-magazine/ask-father/what-does-it-really-mean-to-offer-it-up/.

131. Williams, N. *This is happiness.* New York: Bloomsbury Publishing; 2019, 122.

132. Brody, B. Arteriosclerosis: Your arteries age by age. *WebMD*. December 23, 2013. https://www.webmd.com/heart-disease/features/atherosclerosis-your-arteries-age-by-age.

133. What is osteoarthritis? Osteoarthritis (OA). https://www.versusarthritis.org/about-arthritis/conditions/osteoarthritis/.

134. American Lung Association; 2022. Lung capacity and aging. https://www.lung.org/lung-health-diseases/how-lungs-work/lung-capacity-and-aging.

135. Osteoporosis: Causes. National Health Service, U.K. https://www.nhs.uk/conditions/osteoporosis/causes/.

136. Preserve your muscle mass. Harvard Health Publishing. February 19, 2016. https://www.health.harvard.edu/staying-healthy/preserve-your-muscle-mass.

137. Skelton, D. Explainer: Why does our balance get worse as we grow older? *The Conversation*. October 8, 2015. https://theconversation.com/explainer-why-does-our-balance-get-worse-as-we-grow-older-48197.

138. hear-it.org. Age related hearing loss—presbyacusis. https://www.hear-it.org/Age-related-hearing-loss.

139. How does your vision change with age? Optical Masters. https://www.optical-masters.com/vision-change-age/.

140. Schmidt, S. Americans' views flipped on gay rights. How did minds change so quickly? *Washington Post*. June 7, 2019.

141. Charlesworth, T.E.S., & Banaji, M.R. Do implicit attitudes and beliefs change over the long-term? https://www.umass.edu/employmentequity/sites/default/files/WhatWorks1_Do Implicit Attitudes and Beliefs Change Over Time.pdf.

142. AAMC. Physician Specialty Data Reports from 2008 to 2020. Association of American Medical Colleges. February 2, 2021. https://www.aamc.org/data-reports/data/2020-physician-specialty-data-report-executive-summary.

143. Broxterman, M.P. Physician statistics summary (1970 –1999). Pinnacle Health Group; 2000. https://www.phg.com/2000/01/physician-statistics-summary/.

144. Law school rankings by female enrollment. *Enjuris*. https://www.enjuris.com/students/law-school-women-enrollment-2020.html.

145. Share of lawyers in the U.S. in 2020, by gender. *Statista*. https://www.statista.com/statistics/1086790/share-lawyers-united-states-gender/.

146. Short history of women in the law. *LawCrossing*. May 21, 2013. https://www.lawcrossing.com/article/900014530/A-Short-History-of-Women-in-the-Law/.

147. Belton, D. A generation of American men give up on college: "I just feel lost!" *The Wall Street Journal*. September 6, 2021.

148. Bachelor's, master's, and doctor's degrees conferred by postsecondary institutions, by sex of student and discipline division: 2016-17. Table 318.30. National Center for Education Statistics (2019). https://nces.ed.gov/programs/digest/d18/tables/dt18_318.30.asp.

149. Davidson, J.D., & Widman, T. The effect of group size on interfaith marriage among Catholics. *Journal for the Scientific Study of Religion*. 2002;41(3;December), 399.

150. Davidson & Widman.

151. Goodstein, L. Poll shows major shift in identity of U.S. Jews. *The New York Times*. October 1, 2013.

152. JRank. Interfaith marriage: Prevalence. *Marriage and family encyclopedia*. https://family.jrank.org/pages/897/Interfaith-Marriage-Prevalence.html.

153. Stone, L. Promise and peril: The history of American religiosity and its recent decline. American Enterprise Institute. April 30, 2020. https://www.aei.org/research-products/report/promise-and-peril-the-history-of-american-religiosity-and-its-recent-decline/.

154. Alba, R., Levy, M., & Myers, D. (2021). The myth of a majority-minority America. *The Atlantic*. June 13, 2021. https://www.theatlantic.com/ideas/archive/2021/06/myth-majority-minority-america/619190/

155. Gannon, M. Race is a social construct, scientists argue. *Scientific American*. February 5, 2016. https://www.scientificamerican.com/article/race-is-a-social-construct-scientists-argue/.

156. Tavernise, S., Mzezewa, T., & Heyward, G. Behind the surprising jump in multiracial Americans: Several theories. *The New York Times*. August 13, 2021. https://www.nytimes.com/2021/08/13/us/census-multiracial-identity.html.

157. Tavernise, S., & Gabeloff, R. (2021). Census shows sharply growing numbers of Hispanic, Asian and multiracial Americans. *The New York Times*. August 12, 2021.

158. Tavernise, Mzezewa, & Heyward.

159. Brooks, D. How racist is America? *The New York Times*. July 23, 2021.

160. Tavernise, Mzezewa, & Heyward.
161. Hershfield, H.E. Future self-continuity: How conceptions of the future self-transform intertemporal choice. *Annals of the New York Academy of Science.* October 24, 2011. https://doi.org/10.1111/j.1749-6632.2011.06201.x
162. Hershfield.
163. Neugarten, B.L., Moore, J.W., & Lowe, J.C. Age norms, age constraints and adult socialization. *American Journal of Sociology.* 1965;70(6; May), 70.
164. Ferraro, K.F. The time of our lives: Recognizing the contributions of Mannheim, Neugarten, and Riley to the study of aging. *The Gerontologist.* 2014; 54(1; February), 131. https://doi.org/10.1093/geront/gnt048.
165. Ferraro.
166. Addams, J. *Twenty years at Hull House.* New York: Macmillan; 1911, 156.
167. Addams, 157.
168. Klinenberg, E. *Going solo: The extraordinary rise and surprising appeal of living alone.* New York: Penguin Press; 2013, 3–4.
169. Klinenberg, p. 13.
170. Klinenberg, p. 6.
171. Klinenberg, pp. 17–18.
172. Christensen, C.M., Grossman, J.H., & Hwang, J. *The innovators prescription: A disruptive solution for healthcare.* New York: McGraw-Hill; 2009, 158.
173. Christensen, Grossman, & Hwang, 152.
174. Christensen, Grossman, & Hwang, 150.
175. STOP (Strategies to Overcome and Prevent) Obesity Alliance. Fast facts: The cost of obesity. George Washington University. 2020. https://stop.publichealth.gwu.edu/fast-facts/costs-of-obesity
176. Klinenberg, E. Palaces for the people: How social infrastructure can help fight inequality, polarization, and the decline of civic life. New York: Crown; 2018, 1–7.
177. de Tocqueville, A. *Democracy in America.* Wordsworth Classics of World Literature; 1998 (originally published 1835), 215.
178. Harrison, R.P. The prophet of envy. *New York Review of Books.* December 21, 2018, https://www.nybooks.com/articles/2018/12/20/rene-girard-prophet-envy/.
179. Haven, C.L. *Evolution of desire: A life of René Girard.* East Lansing, MI: Michigan State University Press; 2018, 53.
180. Kurp, P. He knew the reason we fight. Mecosta, MI: Russell Kirk Center for Cultural Renewal; August 19, 2018. https://kirkcenter.org/reviews/he-knew-the-reason-we-fight/.
181. Christakis, N.A., & Fowler, J.H. Connected. New York, Hachette Book Group. 2009, 81.
182. Christakis & Fowler, p. 28.
183. McCamant, K., & Durrett, C. *Cohousing: A contemporary approach to housing ourselves.* Berkeley, CA: Ten Speed Press; 1994.
184. Singh, P. (2021). Nextdoor to go public in $4.3 billion SPAC merger as CEO looks toward expansion. *CNBC.* July 6, 2021. https://www.cnbc.com/2021/07/06/nextdoor-to-go-public-in-4point3-billion-spac-merger-as-ceo-looks-toward-expansion.html.
185. Burstein, D.D. (2013) *Fast future: How the millennial generation is shaping our world.* Boston: Beacon Press; xvii.

186. Burstein, p. 15.
187. Mead, M. *Culture and commitment: A study of the generation gap.* Garden City, NY: Natural History Press; 1970.
188. Putnam, R.D. *Bowling alone: The collapse and revival of American community.* New York: Simon and Schuster; 2000.
189. Dunkelman, M.J. *The vanishing neighbor: The transformation of American community.* New York: W.W. Norton and Company; 2014.

Index

n indicates note.

243